王鳳儀
十二字薪傳

TWELVE CHARACTERS
A TRANSMISSION OF
WANG FENGYI'S TEACHINGS

ALSO BY SABINE WILMS

The Divine Farmer's Classic of Materia Medica
神農本草經 *Shén Nóng Běncǎo Jīng*

Venerating the Root:
Sun Simiao's *Bei Ji Qian Jin Yao Fang*,
volume 5 on Pediatrics ✦ Parts One and Two

Let the Radiant Yang Shine Forth:
Lectures on Virtue by Liu Yousheng

王鳳儀
十二字薪傳

TWELVE CHARACTERS
A TRANSMISSION OF
WANG FENGYI'S TEACHINGS

TRANSLATION BY
SABINE WILMS, PhD

HAPPY GOAT PRODUCTIONS
CORBETT, OREGON • USA

Copyright © 2014 by Sabine Wilms

All rights reserved.
No part of this book may be reproduced in any form
without written permission from the publisher.

PUBLISHED IN THE UNITED STATES OF AMERICA

ISBN 978-0-9913429-6-9

All artwork by Sunjae Lee
www.fermatawellness.com

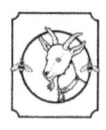

Published by Happy Goat Productions
Corbett, Oregon ▪ USA

For more information and to purchase
other works by Sabine Wilms, visit our website:
www.HappyGoatProductions.com

In the spirit of *xiao*:
unconditional love, service,
and gratitude for our
parents and elders.

CONTENTS

Foreword   ix
Preface   xiii
Acknowledgements   xxv

第一節十二字薪傳
Chapter One:
A Transmission in Twelve Characters   5

第二節三界是人的來蹤
Chapter Two: The Three Realms Are the
Ancestral Footprints that Humans Arrive With   13

第三節三界分清
Chapter Three: A Clear Distinction
Between the Three Realms   19

第四節清三界
Chapter Four: Making the Three Realms Pure   25

第五節三界和三教
Chapter Five: The Three Realms and the Three Teachings   33

第六節三性
Chapter Six: The Three Kinds of Human Nature   41

第七節三命
Chapter Seven: The Three Kinds of Destiny   47

第八節三身
Chapter Eight: The Three Kinds of Body   55

第九節橫超三界
Chapter Nine: Directly Transcending the Three Realms   63

第十節五行性
Chapter Ten: The Five Elements in the Inner Nature — 69

第十一節五行性識別法
Chapter Eleven: How to Differentiate the
Five Elements in the Inner Nature — 83

第十二節心界五行
Chapter Twelve: The Five Elements in the
Realm of the Heart — 89

第十三節身界五行
Chapter Thirteen: The Five Elements in the
Realm of the Body — 95

第十四節五行相生
Chapter Fourteen: The Five Elements
Engendering Each Other — 101

第十五節五行相克
Chapter Fifteen: The Five Elements Overpowering
Each Other — 111

第十六節五行逆運
Chapter Sixteen: The Five Elements Moving Counterflow — 121

第十七節五行圓轉
Chapter Seventeen: Bringing the Five Elements Full Circle — 129

第十八節家庭五行定位
Chapter Eighteen: The Positions of the
Five Elements in the Family — 141

第十九節四大界
Chapter Nineteen: The Four Great Realms — 151

第二十節一串之道
Chapter Twenty: The Dao in a Single String of Beads — 163

Appendix of Key Terms: Pinyin, Chinese, English — 169

FOREWORD

Chinese medicine broadly describes the causes of disease in three major categories – interior causes, exterior causes, and neither interior nor exterior causes. Interior causes are the seven affects of fear, fright, grief, sorrow, worry, joy, and anger. Exterior causes are the environmental disease evils of wind, cold, dryness, dampness, fire, and summerheat. Neither interior nor exterior causes include just about everything else, such as dietary irregularity, sleep patterns, physical trauma, and others. When these three causes of disease are taught to all new Chinese medicine students, there is rarely a discussion about what problems are easy to treat and what are difficult. Often, the more exotic-sounding problems of wind and cold or problems such as bad diets grab a new student's attention. However, most clinicians quite early in their practice come to realize that problems such as wind or diet are easy problems. That which is really the most difficult to deal with are problems of the affects, in other words, problems of the Heart.

For example, clinicians often counsel patients on dietary change. Changing a diet can be a profound thing, and it is at the same time one of the easiest and the hardest of things to change. In theory, it is easy to drastically alter one's health by simply eating differently. All you have to do is put something different in the mouth and diet change is done. However, diet change is one of the hardest to accomplish because people have emotional attachment to eating certain things, or emotional patterns of eating. Thus, while the diet itself is easy to change, the person's Heart is not. Clearly problems of the Heart-mind can be deeply entrenched and can profoundly affect health on all levels.

The early classics of Chinese medicine agree with this assessment. The eighth chapter of the *Huang Di Nei Jing Su Wen*, the Discourse on the Hidden Canons in the Numinous Orchid (*Ling Lan Mi Dian Lun*), likens the Heart, or more accurately the Heart-mind, to the enlightened sovereign, the *jun zhu* (君主). The sum totality of consciousness and our ability to interact with the outside world, including especially other people around us, is what emanates from the Heart. In the *Su Wen* this is called the *shen ming* (神明), the Brilliance of Spirit. The rest of the chapter continues with a description of the other internal organs. However, the end of the chapter returns to the core question of Chinese medicine – what is really at the root of health, wellbeing, and longevity? Qi Bo tells us that the Heart is this root. He says that if the sovereign (i.e., the Heart) is in a state of illumination and enlightenment, then all under its direction will be at peace (故主明則下安). Likewise, if the Heart is not sound, then all the organs are in danger and disaster is soon to follow.

When Chinese medicine came West, Western practitioners of the medicine soon realized the veracity of the Heart's central role in our states of health. They also saw, like many of us still see, that needles or herbs alone are often inadequate in dealing with really shifting a patient's deep-seated habitual emotional patterns. Even in colloquial Chinese there are sayings to this effect. For example, "disease of the heart is difficult to treat (心病難醫)," and "disease of the heart has never been treated with medicine (心病從來無藥醫)." The best way to deal with the Heart is to work with it directly, through the mind and affects – "diseases of the heart must be treated in the heart (i.e., diseases of the heart can only be treated by working with the mind) (心病還用心藥醫)."

Since most Western practitioners of Asian medicines lacked language facility or time spent living or studying in Asia, they naturally tried to graft Western modes of psychology onto Chinese medicine to compensate for the need for a method of working with Heart. One of my own early frustrations with practicing Chinese medicine was the lack of authentic indigenous Asian methods of working with the Heart that could be implemented in a modern clinical setting. I truly believed, and still believe, that since Asian medicine grew in the soil of traditional Asian culture and philosophy, it is preferable to first explore authentic methods of working with the Heart-mind before randomly conflating Chinese medicine with modern Western modes of psychotherapy, which are sometimes quite at odds.

As the field of Chinese medicine and even Asian studies advances, more and more material has come to the West, including indigenous methods of using Heart to treat Heart. Today, methods such as Buddhist approaches to psychology or Japanese Naikan or Morita therapy are being taught and utilized clinically in the Western world, and there are numerous Western language books that explore these methods. This new book translated by Dr. Sabine Wilms presents yet another authentic Asian method of working with the Heart, the teachings of the Confucian healer Wang Fengyi.

Wang Fengyi's method is different from those others just mentioned in that it is based on the classical Chinese theory of the Five Phases (also known as Five Elements). Wang Fengyi's enlightenment was in part his ability to see clearly the complexity of human relationships and human emotions through the lens of the Five Phases, in a much more complete and detailed way than had previously been done in Chinese medicine. Using this understanding, he developed a way to understand the deep roots of disease and how they are directly linked to the Heart-mind. The good master Wang paints a clear path to health and happiness that is found by looking within and honestly evaluating our own lives. This is empowering in that it places our health in our own hands. Wang also teaches us that we choose whether we live in heaven or hell, right now, in our current life.

What is particularly compelling for me as a practitioner of Chinese medicine is that the theories presented in this text are those that can be easily incorporated into Chinese medicine practice precisely because they use the same language of Chinese medicine. Wang's astute observation of the different Five Phase emotional types, which includes observations of body morphology as well as typical emotional and behavioral patterns, is remarkably detailed and amazingly accurate in the clinic. While Wang was familiar with the various religions of his day, he advocated that they all contain similar goals. Thus, his own system is presented as a practical non-sectarian secular method of working with the Heart that can be followed by any person of any creed.

I believe this book will make a significant contribution to the field of Chinese medicine in the Western world, and as such Dr. Wilms has done us all a great service in bringing this translation to print. My hope is that the material presented here will also spread beyond practitioners of Chinese medicine and in doing so help alleviate suffering and the cause of suffering for all beings under the sky.

Dr. Henry McCann (馬爾博)
Written during Autumn Equinox In the Jia Wu Year, 2014
New Jersey, USA

PREFACE

"You want happiness? It is right here within your reach."

So begins the "Transmission of 12 Characters" this concise, compact record of Wang Fengyi's teachings you hold in your hand. These are not just words, for he proceeds to tell us how to reach it, providing specific, powerful and proven directives, that if applied sincerely, will penetrate the fog of your old ways of operating and change your life. Guaranteed. These teachings are given for the sake of "exalting the human Nature" and "expressing the Heavenly Nature to its fullest potential." This book is healing medicine - medicine for the "Heart".

What are the words that would truly honor such a purpose? I have grappled with this since first reading the draft, spinning a bit in circles, until a wise friend helped me see – there were no words that could fully honor this work for what is being offered is beyond the limitations of language. And so, my sincerest intent in this preface is to encourage you, the reader, to begin experiencing these life affirming teachings – not just read them – but rather live them, letting them breathe their wisdom into you in a way that just might radically shift your life, allowing the magnificence that you already are to fully emerge.

I think back to how my own life has changed, and continues to, since first being introduced to these Confucian-based teachings of Wang Fengyi as found in the Shan Ren Dao system. From the moment I first heard a dear friend describing his experience with this work I was mesmerized – pulled in as if by an inextricable force – everything in me said "yes." My response was not just to the words I was hearing, but to the change I saw in front of me in this man whom I knew so well. Something had definitely happened in China when he experienced this work. What were these teachings that focused on "healing the heart" and in the process, healing on the physical level as well, often in profound and seemingly "miraculous" ways?

A year later when the opportunity arose for Westerners to attend a Shan Ren Dao retreat in China for the first (and only) time to date, there was no question, I was going. I had no idea what to expect. I had already missed the informational interview process. I simply arrived. It was the only thing I could do.

I wondered why such a strong pull. Having been a "seeker" for many years, surely I had experienced enough exposure to different systems, theories and approaches to self-growth by that time in my life. With a doctoral degree in Naturopathic medicine and a master's degree in Chinese medicine, I also had significant exposure to diverse approaches to healing and health. And yet, there was something missing. While many systems gave voice to a "holistic" approach to medicine, one that included the body, mind, and spirit, rarely did I see that effectively move from the theoretical realms into actual clinical practice. I was seeking something to bridge that gap.

Could these teachings provide that "something" – a substantial, accessible and well proven approach to health that fundamentally impacts not only the way we think, live and experience our lives, but also the material level of the physical body? From what I had heard the answer was yes. Curious and excited, yet with a dose of caution and skepticism, I arrived in China.

Now, here I was on day two in a remote monastery - my body hot, aching all over, fluids streaming from my nose and a blazing sore throat. Was this the "detox" of emotions to which this system referred? Could this be my body releasing toxins I didn't even know I had? And if so, initiated by what - the few minutes I spent speaking of my appreciation of my ancestors? According to the Shan Ren Dao system this is exactly what was happening. As you open with gratitude to your ancestors for the gift of this sacred body that has allowed you the opportunity for life itself, you connect to the Original Source Qi (energy) and realign with the heavens. As pure Qi increases in your body in this aligned state, toxins begin to leave. Each person's physical expression, including their toxin release, in this detailed system based on the Chinese five phase elements, provides a specific clue to the emotions that have sat inside, non-integrated, and, over time damaging the health of the organs and body.

I became increasingly excited when, a day later, mild to moderate kidney pain that had plagued me periodically for the past 10 years suddenly lifted. Even more astounding was the disappearance of the constant vulnerability and aching in the vertebra/disc in my cervical (neck) spine. It was the lingering residual from a significant car accident 13 years earlier and was something I assumed would simply be there for life. That was pre-Wang Fengyi and Shan Ren Dao. Suddenly that too - gone. Each morning I would check. Disbelieving, and perhaps even daring it to return, I would drop my heels down hard in the morning qigong practice, creating the vibration up my spine which had been intolerable the previous 13 years. That had my attention, the pain was truly gone.

Even more than the physical however, were the changes I noticed inside me relative to others. I first became aware of a streaming inner voice of judgment, and then noticed its quieting. I thought my relationship with my parents was really good, and yet in the retreat something unexpected occurred. I became aware of a block in my heart, a distinct contraction sitting there. In time, as I applied the teachings and continued to allow my feelings, reactions and behaviors to surface, even those most uncomfortable, a distinct sensation of expansion and opening began in my heart. It was as if my heart became available for a deeper, more joyous connection. This is the power of this "Heart medicine" and we need it as much now, perhaps even more, than in Wang Fengyi's time 150 years ago.

We are social beings, designed to be in relationship. The yearning to be truly seen, accepted and loved sits at our deepest core. When our relationships are out of order, we become stressed and stress is increasingly recognized as the leading cause of illness in the West. In developed countries we have become stressed nations of chronic disease and for that, western medicine has little to offer. Wang Fengyi foresaw this development. He recognized, even in his time, the primary cause of disease had shifted from malnourishment, poor sanitation and infectious disease to illnesses of disconnection, suffered as people focused increasingly on the material to the detriment of relationship. He spoke of the "terror" in his heart as he predicted the expanding "battlefields" and "chaos" that would reign should this fight for material things exceed the care of and love for each other. We are there.

We have increasingly become individual islands, alone, fiercely independent, and yet yearning for the connection that is the natural state of being for our Heart. The rampant use of cell phones further amplifies our distance. Just walk into any restaurant, a formerly sacred time for people to connect and "unplug", and watch the number of people speaking on their cell phones rather than to the person in front of them. Mother Teresa cautioned us on this as well, stating:

> The greatest disease in the West today is not TB or leprosy; it is being unwanted, unloved, and uncared for. We can cure physical diseases with medicine, but the only cure for loneliness, despair, and hopelessness is love. There are many in the world who are dying for a piece of bread but there are many more dying for a little love. The poverty in the West is a different kind of poverty—it is not only a poverty of loneliness but also of spirituality. There's a hunger for love, as there is a hunger for God.

Most illness in our western culture is indeed illness of the Heart and we are looking for answers – hoping to counter this distress of disconnection. Books and movies on empowerment and manifestation and the interconnectedness of all things have flourished.

Wang Fengyi offers a solution, cutting straight to the chase and telling us unequivocally, if we are to live lives that honor our magnificence and the fullness of our human potential it is our Heart that needs rectifying. In this context, we refer to the larger Heart spoken of in Wisdom teachings throughout time – that which is an organ of inner alignment, complete ability and connection. This Heart allows us to be guided by and aligned with our divinity while having a human experience.

How do we do it?

In just twelve characters he delivers condensed wisdom and guidance on what a human is and how to reveal our numinous True Nature. It is the "Being Human 101" course we all need (and likely never received).

What are these twelve characters?

The first three characters, Inner Nature, Heart and Body, similar to the Spirit, Mind, and Body analogy common in the West, describe what it is to be human. They also describe what it is to be part of an unbroken lineage receiving gifts from our ancestors as well as old, restrictive emotional operating patterns.

He reminds us first and foremost we all arrive endowed with a Heavenly Inner Nature of pure light. This Inner Nature is flawless. It knows only love. There is nothing we need to improve upon or do, it is already perfect. When we are aligned with it and led by it, we mature fully into ourselves as humans. We also come with a pure Heart, as mentioned earlier, this organ of alignment which connects us to the divine and our creative abilities. The third realm from which we operate is the material. We arrive with a body vessel, perfectly designed to carry us around in this earthly realm.

In this system, we start with the recognition of our purity and perfection. Connecting to this provides the light and courage to begin to see where we operate in ways seemingly counter to this nature, erecting instead lives of unhappy existence. Why do so many of us live like this when we are already perfect? Wang Fengyi tells us it is because we also arrive imprinted with *"bingxing"* – specific, habitual, outdated ways of reacting that show up, not only in our lives, but have been part of the operating system of our lineage, often for generations. Much as clouds in the sky can completely hide the sun, these *bingxing* cover our inner light. We forget it exists. We forget what we are.

We know we are operating from this *bingxing* when we are stuck – repeating the same pattern over and over- the same arguments, the same feelings, the same life experiences (even if under different apparent covers). It is that part of us which responds with anger, hatred, blame, irritation or annoyance to others. These clouds get thicker when we allow our emotions to rule us, giving free reign to our selfish desires and physical addictions. Wang Fengyi recognized the incredible power and destructive force of these states. Many other ancient traditions have recognized the same. I heard a traditional Maori healer speak about the way we have empowered emotions to the point of creating a "fifth being" in this world. And rather than being masters of our emotions, this emotional "being" masters us - dictating how we feel, move, breathe, act and relate. This is living from the *bingxing*. It is not that we are to live without emotions or deny or suppress them. That is just as dangerous and paradoxically, the suppressed emotions run us as much, or more, as those expressed excessively. When our Heavenly Nature and True Heart are in the driver's seat, emotions come into balance where they can be wonderful informers and resources. When the emotional being or *bingxing* is in the driver seat, havoc reigns and our "reality" becomes contracted and rife with jealousy, fear, doubt, unworthiness, anger and many other disconnecting emotions. That is the "reality" of our *bingxing*. There exists another reality.

Wang Fengyi joins other great sages, Wisdom teachers and many of the traditional spiritual paths, which have in their own way throughout the ages, spoken of the need to change our perceptual operating system. They call us to make the shift from the habitual, reactive, "small" self to the large "Self" – where our Inner Heavenly Nature, our Heart and our Body are aligned as one and we are able to manifest the fullness of our humanity. Each highlights specific practices to reach the goal; the end goal is the same. Wang Fengyi makes it very clear however, this is not a religious path, "but rather honors the (chosen) religious paths as the "right" path for each."

Unique to this system, Wang Fengyi uses the body symptoms and illness to inform where the toxic nonintegrated emotions are clouding our Inner Nature. One of the challenges with any path that directs you inward is the difficulty in truly seeing yourself, your purity as well as the *bingxing*. He recognized the body doesn't lie – it can't. If your Inner Nature is clouded, your

Body will be clouded and vice versa. For Wang Fengyi there was no differentiation between physical, emotional and spiritual toxicity. Acting from obstructive emotions in any of the three realms immediately translates into physical poisons. It is a "law". If signs of hatred are showing up on the external – through your red rash, itchiness, fiery eruptions or heart symptoms, there is hatred toxicity on the inside. You then know to look for the hatred that is still harbored toward another (and ultimately toward yourself). Your symptoms become a precious guide directing you to the source. He himself suffered from a life-threatening abdominal abscess for over a decade that spontaneously healed overnight when he recognized that despite being known as someone who lived a life of genuine respect and care for others, especially his elders, on the inner he was filled with blame towards those he viewed as not living from his same values. This awareness of his own hypocrisy, followed immediately by a firm commitment to stop all blaming, produced an immediate and dramatic physical healing. It was a pivotal moment in his life, leading to what was to become this complete system of healing and opening to life's potential.

The next five characters describe this link between emotions and physical illness, as well as family relationships and the five phase elements of Chinese medicine. They take the philosophy of the Three Realms of the Inner Nature, Heart and Body and ground it in visible specifics of everyday life. There is both a "yang" aspect (our natural emotional expression when we are aligned with our truth and connection) and a "yin" aspect (that emotion that arises when we are operating from old patterns of separation) associated with each element. Through exploring these five elements and how they move and interact, we begin to see our own specific patterns of responding (or reacting) to experiences in the world. These patterns, along with their specific physical correlations provide detailed descriptions allowing us to see where we are stuck within ourselves and in our relationships.

And, as we become aware of these patterns AND begin to deeply feel the impact of our behaviors on others, the toxins begin to disperse. The ways in which this toxicity releases from your body also varies depending, for example, on whether the toxin is more of the hating type or more of the blaming type or more of the judgment type. This then provides additional clues to further direct inward reflection and exploration.

As these patterns clear, we naturally express the "yang" aspects of the five elements within. We begin to live lives led by empathy, integrity selflessness, wisdom and respect. We move from hatred and attempting to withdraw and protect our heart, to connection. We choose integrity and self-responsibility over blame. We respect and honor the differing paths of others where once we were irritated or critical. We surrender the need to be superior or all-knowing in exchange for the wisdom that arises from humility. We extend compassion, choosing to see from another's perspective versus treating them with anger. It is not that we are forcing ourselves to act as a "good" person, rather we are simply being in our natural expression. As Wang Fengyi tells us: "When the Realm of the Inner Nature is clear, the person has no ill temper. When the Realm of the Heart is clear, the person has no selfish desires. When the Realm of the Body is clear, the person has no vile addictions." Then our true radiance shines forth. This he tells us, is the route to find happiness and heaven here on earth. We have choice. This brings us to the final four characters that delineate four distinct "worlds" or ways of existing here on earth. We get to choose to which we will aspire and commit as we set our feet upon that path to our future.

How do we do it?
In his direct, pragmatic way Wang Fengyi offers simple guidance: *"Looking for the positive in others opens the road to paradise in Heaven; acknowledging your wrongs closes the gates to hell on Earth."*

This is the path in a nutshell. If you follow this simple advice, your relationships and your life will change. Of this he assures us and tens of thousands of people have born witness to the veracity of this approach.

Where do we start applying this simple guidance in creating harmony, peace, and "heaven" while here on earth?
He points us to those relationships closest to us, those in which we also tend to "act out" the most. This is the place to start. Being "good" out in the world while having emotional outbursts at home with those most beloved

is destructive and thickens the obstructive cloud layers. This is world work. As we heal these relationships and more harmony is created in our family, it ripples out to impact our community, our country and the very world in which we live. Wang Fengyi, true to his Confucian roots, recognized that changing the world requires starting with the center - our families.

How can you get the most from this book?

These teachings are pure gold. Like other ancient wisdom teachings, they are a profound gift whose message is timeless, as relevant now as we seek the direction of our heart, as they were 150 years ago. To get the most from this book, there are a few useful things to keep in mind.

First, this book is not designed as a stand-alone entry book. These teachings can only be known experientially and are traditionally transmitted orally, either individually or in a retreat immersion setting. Contained within these pages are a record of the entry, middle and advanced aspects of this system. As such this book will be difficult to access for people with no prior exposure to these teachings. This is especially true of the later chapters of the five element section on engendering, overpowering and counterflow. Those sections are for advanced practitioners. If you are new to these teachings, you might want to skip those for now. In the traditional immersion retreats that information is not covered and is not necessary for this system to work its magic.

Despite how it may appear on initial reading however, the system is simple – do not be fooled by the apparent complexity of the theory. It was designed as an accessible healing system for rural, illiterate peasants in Northern China. Wang Fengyi himself was an illiterate peasant. The basic concepts are straight-forward, easily grasped and yet far-reaching in their depth and impact. Pull out these pearls and sit with them. Let them instruct you. Let the rest go.

Second, in her translation Dr. Sabine Wilms has stayed impeccably true to the original content rather than modifying it to make it more "user" friendly and thus increase the risk of inaccuracies. As a result, some of the language can only be understood within the context of a specific century and culture.

Rather than be deterred by some of the language, I encourage you observe your resistance, as well as expand around it, allowing the deep meaning and truth to emerge. You can also just skip it for now and return later. Each time you reread this material you will understand more.

Third, I have noticed in the West there can be a tendency for people to interpret these teachings as instruction to be "good" or be "better." In our culture, that often translates as suppressing emotions, not speaking your truth, attempting to please others and other ways of "disappearing." That is absolutely not what these teachings are about. In fact, on the contrary, they are about being impeccably responsible. They are about becoming masters of our own ship and destiny. When we blame it takes us from our center – we become victims, we lose our agency in the world and we become small. As we instead follow the guidance to become responsible for our emotions and our ways of relating, in time we discover we feel more ourselves now than ever previously. As the habitual patterning begins to fall away, we act, speak and think from the deeper core of who we are. What does that mean? It means we are empowered to speak and live from a deeper truth, to live a life of alignment and integrity inside and out – to live as we were designed. And, in that there is a natural "goodness" – one that equally honors our existence as well as another's. It is not selfish, but rather generous and more abundant than we can imagine.

Fourth, and most importantly, these teachings are experiential. This material can only be known experientially. As Wang Fengyi tells us, no path exists unless you walk it. You must find a way to put it into practice. Apply each section before moving on or read the entire book once through and then come back and start again, moving more slowly and applying each section.

What about the Shan Ren Dao immersion retreats?

In 2011, we had the remarkable opportunity to bring these teachings to the west in the traditional immersion retreat format passed on by Wang Fengyi and my teacher Liu Shanren. It became clear from the very first retreat that this "Heart medicine" transcends cultural boundaries and has a significant impact for those experiencing it in the United States. We have since continued to hold two-week immersion Shan Ren Dao retreats annually in the

Pacific Northwest. While our sample group is still small, individual reports on physical healings have ranged from the resolution of chronic pain, to normalization of blood work, to being cancer-free, and in one case to the disappearance of tumors as verified on scans. Even more significant than the physical reports are the changes in relationships and the experience of life itself.

However you first access this material, whether through retreats or books or another individual, it is the beginning, not the completion of the journey. The teachings provide specific guidance and practical tools to mine life's challenges and utilize them for growth - tools to call forth your true virtues, tools to release these old toxic states, tools that stand by you as you begin to negotiate the world in new ways and tools that support connection and health as opposed to separation and dis-ease. The wonderful thing is you don't need to understand all the theory or be psychologically astute. Simply apply the tools.

One of the wondrously paradoxical things I have seen in this brilliant work, is through the focus on the outer we return to the self. As we change the way we relate to others, it automatically begins to influence the way we relate to ourselves. Your relationship to yourself begins to heal. Just last week a retreat participant from several years ago called me to say, "Something has happened. For the first time in my life I realized yesterday my perceptions of what others think of me have been completely wrong my entire life". She then continued in a tone of absolute awe "I actually just discovered I am 'ok'…In fact, I really like myself." Yesterday, another told me "For the first time in my life I feel my relationships now are of such high integrity and honesty. I feel so filled with love and gratitude. This is what I have yearned for my entire life."

If you have doubt, try one "simple" thing. For the next 8 weeks simply "do not blame." Do not blame anyone. Do not blame others. Do not blame yourself.

Such a simple thing and yet it will unfold you, layer by layer, beginning to peel away places you have disempowered yourself. As blame leaves – we arrive – back in our center – increasingly living the lives of integrity to which we aspire. But do not take my word for it. Then it simply becomes a theory soon to be regulated to the back recesses of the mind as so many others. No, just do it. I challenge you. I encourage you. I implore you. As Wang Fengyi teaches us, "Spare no effort to put it into practice." Then write me on how your life is different. As the sage tells us "The more we walk it, the more we prove it; the more faith we have, the more solid it becomes."

That this book is available in English comes from the contributions of many. My deepest gratitude to Liu Shanren for dedicating his life to disseminating these teachings to others for over half a century and his willingness to open the door to people from the West. Dr. Heiner Fruehauf and Dr. Liu Lihong in their tireless commitment to seeking out the hidden gems found within the classical teachings, discovered this path and, along with Abbott Mingchan, moved heaven and earth to first make it available to those outside of China. This translation would not exist were it not for Dr. Sabine Wilms. Following her participation in a Shan Ren Dao retreat she committed to bringing her extensive professional translation skills to bear in making these teachings available to a wider English speaking audience. Her integrity and firmness in translating the original meaning as closely as possible is priceless. This is the second book of these teachings she has translated. A special thanks to Laurie Regan who recognizing the importance of this work, has determinedly found a way to make it available to students in the Classical Chinese Medicine Programs at the National University of Natural Medicine and who has unwaveringly supported me and the Shan Ren Dao retreats. Without the assistants who have so lovingly and generously given of their time none of this would have been possible. Perhaps most of all, it is the exuberant response of those who have participated in the English speaking retreats and continue to walk the path and expand its dissemination in the West, that has driven the creation of this book. Thank you.

In closing let me simply state, "This stuff works."

Tamara Staudt, ND, LAc
Faculty, College of Classical Chinese Medicine
National University of Natural Medicine,
Portland, Oregon, USA

ACKNOWLEDGEMENTS

There is no greater gift in today's world than to heal the relationship with our parents, to reconnect us to where we came from, to remind us of the true nature of existence, which is infinite love. And that is what Wang Fengyi's teachings do.

The insights expressed in this book have completely changed the way I look at and live in the world. Not a day passes without my being touched in some way by the gift that the experience of the Shan Ren Dao retreat and my subsequent translation work with this material has been for me. The seemingly simple instruction "Do Not Blame!" challenges me daily to turn my gaze inward, take responsibility for walking my Dao, and learn how to live in my Heavenly Nature.

This book is an attempt to share that gift with you, our readers. Read it slowly for it contains many gems.

In addition to the people who Tamara Staudt mentions in her beautiful introduction, I would like to thank Renae Rogers and Henry McCann for reviewing the manuscript and, in Henry's case, also for writing a preface and adding clinical comments; Kimberly Reed and Barbara Tada for their labor of love in turning my manuscript into the beautiful book you hold in your hands; and Sunjae Lee for the gorgeous artwork. Lastly, I would like to state the obvious: I wouldn't be who I am and have the skills that allow me to do what I do without my parents' undying love and support. No words can fully express my gratitude to them, and to Wang Fengyi, to my teachers in this work – Liu Lihong, Abbot Ming Chan, Heiner Fruehauf, Laurie Regan, and Tamara Staudt – and to my fellow walkers on the Shan Ren Dao.

Sabine Wilms, PhD
Corbett, Oregon

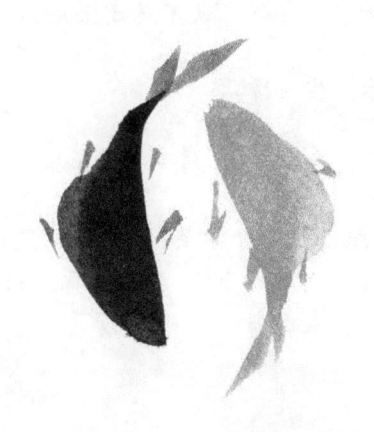

你想快乐么？你就会得到。

人人有无无边罪恶，一一悔便消。

认不是生生智慧水水，找好处生生响亮金金。

认不是胜用用清凉散，找好处胜服暖心心丸。

找好处开了天堂路，认不是闭上地狱门。

观想极乐，尘飞障落。

乐一一乐天堂有个座，愁一一愁地狱游一一游。

不会笑，照着镜子子学笑，笑得比比哭还难看。先是假笑，时间久了，弄假成真，快乐就从心心里里生生出来了。

You want happiness? It is right here, within your reach.

> Humans commit unlimited crimes and evil, but just a single thought of remorse, and these vanish.
>
> Acknowledging your wrongs generates deep wisdom, the virtue of Water; looking for the positive in others generates shining radiance, the virtue of Metal.
>
> To triumph in acknowledging your wrongs, employ the medicine of Clear and Pure Powder; to triumph in looking for the positive in others, take Heart-Warming Pill.[1]
>
> Looking for the positive in others opens the road to paradise in Heaven; acknowledging your wrongs closes the gates to hell on Earth.
>
> By contemplating ultimate bliss, the dust of the world flies off and obstructions melt away.
>
> With an attitude of constant happiness, there is a place for you in Heaven; with an attitude of constant worry, you will travel to hell on Earth.
>
> If you don't know how to laugh, look in the mirror and learn how to do it, even though it may be more awkward than crying. At first, it may be a false laugh, but over time, if you stick with it, pretense becomes reality, and happiness will be born from your heart.

---

[1] Please note that the names "Clear and Pure Powder" and "Heart-Warming Pill" do not refer to actual herbal formulas from the repertory of Chinese medicine but are meant figuratively here, as metaphors for the internal work of self-cultivation.

CHAPTER ONE

十二字薪傳

A Transmission in Twelve Characters

王善人讲的道只有十二个字，就是"性、心、身""木、火、土、金、水""志、意、心、身"。

性、心、身三界是人的来踪，为入世之法；运用木、火、土、金、水五行当人，为应世之法；志、意、心、身四大界是人的去路，为出世之法。会了这十二个字，才能来得明，去得白。性、心、身三界归一，五行圆转，四大界定位，便当体成真，能为圣为贤，成佛做祖。

The Dao that the venerable Wang Fengyi taught consists of only twelve characters: Inner Nature (*xing* 性), Heart (*xin* 心), and Body (*shen* 身); Wood (*mu* 木), Fire (*huo* 火), Earth (*tu* 土), Metal (*jin* 金), and Water (*shui* 水); and Commitment (*zhi* 志), Intention (*yi* 意), Heart (*xin* 心), and Body (*shen* 身).[2]

The Three Realms (*san jie*) – the Inner Nature, Heart, and Body – contain the ancestral footprints that we humans arrive with, the imprinted pattern with which we enter the world. How we use the Five Elements (*wu xing*)[3] – Wood, Fire, Earth, Metal, and Water – in our actions as human beings is the imprinted pattern with which we respond to the world. The Four Great Realms (*si da jie*) – Commitment, Intention, Heart, and Body – are the road to our future, the imprinted pattern with which we exit the world. Only when we master these twelve concepts can we understand where we come from and go to. When the Three Realms (Inner Nature, Heart, and Body) have returned to a state of oneness, when the Five Elements succeed each other in a perfect cycle, and when the Four Great Realms occupy their proper place, then we can manifest our true selves in our present body, act as saints and sages, and then become Buddhas and join the ranks of our esteemed ancestors.

---

2 Throughout this book, we have decided to capitalize key terms that are used in Wang Fengyi's teachings with an added layer of meaning that transcends their common English usage. For a complete list of these terms, see the Appendix to this book, where they are listed with the Chinese character and pinyin pronunciation. While it is admittedly impossible to find a single English word to convey the meaning of a character like *li* 理 (in the following pages translated somewhat awkwardly and untraditionally as "Guidance"), we have chosen this strategy as a lesser of two evils, so as to make Wang Fengyi's teachings as accessible as possible to readers with no background in the Chinese language.

3 In spite of my personal reservations, I have chosen to continue the common English practice of translating *wu xing* 五行 as "Five Elements" because of the popularity of that term and its established use in other English literature on Wang Fengyi's teachings. It is important to note, however, that the Chinese term literally means "Five Movements" and does NOT refer to elements in the sense of basic material constituents but rather to characteristics of movement and directions of change in the continuous transformation of qi. As such, translations like "five dynamic movements" or "five phases" come much closer to the sense of the Chinese term than "five elements."

可惜世人，只注重身外的事物，不注重自己的心性，真是舍本求末。有的人因为不知道不去行；有的人明明知道而不肯实行，得不着其中奥妙，享不着人生幸福，糟蹋了成佛作祖的材料。所以善人说"讲道不离身，打铁不离砧。"我们听了道，得往自己身上归，努力实行，才能得着受用。讲道不往身上归，好象铁匠离开铁砧打铁一样，如何能成呢？

现在的天时是天不爱道、地不爱宝、人不爱情，万教齐发，科学日进。科学越进步，人类越需要以道德为主，才能享受到物质的幸福。人要能各正性命，爱人如己，就不会为争物质而牺牲人命了。世上的人，要全有宗教信仰，各行各道，各做各德，谁也妨碍不着谁，人多福大，道多德大，天堂极乐世界就在眼前了。

How unfortunate that most people only focus on matters outside themselves, instead of on their Heart and Inner Nature! This is indeed a case of "abandoning the root to pursue the tip." Some people, on account of their ignorance of the Dao, fail to walk it; others, however, have a crystal clear understanding of the Dao and yet are unwilling to walk it in practice. As such, they are unable to grasp the subtle mysteries at its center, to enjoy all the blessings and good fortune that human life has to offer, and they ruin the raw material that is their potential for becoming a Buddha and esteemed ancestor. For this reason, the venerable Wang Fengyi said: "When teaching the Dao, do not stray from your personal experience, just as you do not stray from the anvil when forging iron." Once we have heard the Dao, we must turn inward and apply it to our own personal situation, sparing no effort to put it into practice. That is the only way that it will be of any use. If we do not reflect back on our personal experience when teaching the Dao, this is just like a blacksmith who leaves the anvil to forge iron. How can this be effective?

Our modern times are such that Heaven does not begrudge the Dao, Earth does not begrudge its treasures, and humans do not begrudge their feelings. Thousands of teachings are developing side by side, and science is advancing day by day. And yet, the more scientific progress we experience, the greater the need for humanity to let itself be ruled by Dao and by Virtue (as the manifestation thereof),[4] if we are to enjoy our material bounty. We must each individually rectify our Inner Nature (*xing*) and our Destiny (*ming*) and love others as we love ourselves, to avoid sacrificing our lives in the fight over material things. Every person in the world must have religion and faith, each must walk the Dao and practice Virtue, and nobody must hinder another person's progress. Then humanity will be greatly blessed and the Dao will manifest abundantly in Virtue. The Heavenly Paradise and Pure Land[5] will be right before our eyes.

---

4 *Daode*: Literally translated, Dao means simply "Way," the path that shows us where to walk and how to act. From this basic meaning, the term has come to assume a deep significance in Chinese philosophy, in the Confucian context as the way for humans to interact with each other, and in the Daoist context as the cosmic Dao, the Dao of Heaven and Earth. Virtue (*de*) is the manifestation of the Dao in human actions.

5 *Qing tu* 淨土: "Pure Land" is a technical term from Mahayana Buddhism that refers to the celestial realms where Buddhas or bodhisattvas reside.

用不着向外去追求，人人笃行五伦人道，家庭一定和乐。人人有正当职业，国家一定平靖。人人有道德，世界就大同了。如果只知争贪物质，不知爱人，科学愈发达，战场就越扩大，物质越文明，世界就越混乱。不但自己的身命难保，就是性灵也将万劫难复。言念及此，真使人胆战心惊！

佛家说："人身难得，中土难生，大道难闻。"现在大道昌明，各教都把道送在人的眼前，好象山珍海味，都摆在面前，只要你肯吃，就得着了。道研究明白了，还要诚心实行，越行越能证道，越做信心越坚，就能做个顶天立地、继往开来的圣贤，也就能造福人群，立住万古。善人说："道不行，用不着道；德不作，就没有德。"大家应该好好研究研究吧！

There is no use in searching for solutions on the outside. If everybody earnestly walks the human Dao of the Five Relationships,[6] the family will most certainly be harmonious and happy. If everybody has a proper occupation, the country will most certainly be at peace. If everybody has Dao and manifests it in virtuous actions, Great Harmony will rule in the world. But if people only know how to fight over material things and not how to love others, then the more science develops, the more the battlefields will expand, and the more sophisticated material goods become, the more chaos will reign in the world. Not only will it be difficult to protect our own lives, but it will spell disaster for our souls, and it will be difficult to retrieve them. Just reading these words strikes terror into my heart!

Chinese Buddhists have a saying: "It is a rare gift to incarnate in a human body, it is a rare gift to be born in the Middle Kingdom,[7] and it is a rare gift to hear the Great Dao." At present, the Great Dao is shining forth brightly, each religion delivering it straight in front of people's eyes, like a banquet of rare treasures from the mountains and seas arranged right before us. All we have to do to get it is to be willing to open our mouths. After we have studied and comprehended the Dao, we still have to wholeheartedly walk it in practice. The more we walk it, the more we prove it; the more faith we have, the more solid it becomes. In this way, we can become saints of indomitable spirit, holding up Heaven while grounded in Earth. We are also able to do good deeds for the benefit of humanity, standing firmly for eternity. As the venerable Wang Fengyi said: "If you don't walk the Dao, you don't know how to use it. If you do not translate Virtue into action, there simply is no Virtue." Everybody, investigate this topic with great care and attention!

---

6 This is a reference to the five relationships that regulate Chinese society in traditional Confucian thinking: father to son, husband to wife, ruler to ruled, elder brother to younger brother, and friend to friend. To translate these roles into modern life, we can transcend their gender-specific limitations and instead read them as parent to child, life partner to life partner, superior or inferior, older sibling to younger sibling, and friend to friend. The key point is still relevant, namely that these roles are clearly defined and properly fulfilled.

7 Chinese people refer to China as *Zhongguo* 中国, the "Middle Kingdom."

CHAPTER TWO

三界是人的來蹤

The Three Realms Are the
Ancestral Footprints that
Humans Arrive With

人是天地人三界生的。天赋给人的性，地赋给人的命，父母赋给人的身，所以说"三界是人的来踪。"

人的天性是纯阳的，只知为人，不知为己；心是半阴半阳的，所以才有人心（为己）道心（为人）的分别；身体是个胎生物，是纯阴的，所以只知有己，不知有人。

人要性存天理，心存道理，身尽情理。情理足、道理圆，道理足、天理圆，天理足，性光就能圆。明自本心，见自本性，光灼灼、圆陀陀，便是返本归原成道了。王善人说："一个人就是一个天地，一个阴阳，可惜人都不知道。实在说，天地有坏，我性无坏，人比天地还贵重得多呢！天虽至清，没人行道德，不能明真理；地虽得宁，没人开荒垦土，不能自成田园。所以人有操纵天地的能力。"既然明道，知三界是人的来踪，天地虽大，人也不小，就得行道，才是寻宗返本的大路。

As humans, we are born from the Three Realms of Heaven, Earth, and Humanity (*tian di ren san jie*). Heaven bestows on us our Inner Nature (*xing*), Earth bestows on us our Destiny (*ming*), and our parents bestow on us our Body (*shen*). Therefore we say, "The Three Realms are the ancestral footprints that we humans arrive with."

Our Heavenly Nature is pure yang and knows only how to exist for the sake of others, not how to exist for the self. The Heart is half yang and half yin, and we therefore make a distinction between the Human Heart (for the self) and the Dao Heart (for others). The Body, lastly, is a material thing born from a fetus. It is pure yin and therefore knows only of the existence of the self, but not of the existence of others.

As humans, we want to harbor the Ordering Principle of Heaven (*tianli*) in our Inner Nature, to harbor the Ordering Principle of the Dao (*daoli*) in our Heart, and to fully express the Ordering Principle of the Emotions (*qingli*) in our Body. When the Ordering Principle of the Emotions is fulfilled, the Ordering Principle of the Dao comes full circle. When the Ordering Principle of the Dao is fulfilled, the Ordering Principle of Heaven comes full circle. When the Ordering Principle of Heaven is fulfilled, the radiance of our Inner Nature is able to come full circle. When understanding comes from the original Heart and seeing comes from the original Inner Nature, oh what radiant brightness, what a pearl of perfection! Returning to the root and source brings the Dao to fruition. The venerable Wang Fengyi said: "A single person is Heaven and Earth, yin and yang. How unfortunate that people generally do not know this! In reality, Heaven and Earth are flawed, but our Inner Nature is without flaws. So Humanity is far more precious than Heaven and Earth! Even though Heaven is of utmost purity, without Humans to walk the Dao and manifest it in Virtue, it is unable to shed light on its truth. Even though Earth is able to be tranquil, without Humans to open up wilderness and cultivate the land, it cannot become fields and gardens on its own. Humans hence have the capacity to adapt Heaven and Earth to their needs." Now you comprehend the Dao and know that the Three Realms are the ancestral footprints that we humans arrive with. You realize that even though Heaven and Earth are great, Humanity is not small either. Understanding this, you must simply

孔子行忠恕，耶稣行博爱，穆罕默德行仁恕，老子用感应，佛行慈悲。五教教主，全是用善心，行天道。他们都知道身体是个臭皮囊，早晚是要坏的，只有天性，能存万古。所以孔子主张"杀身成仁"；耶稣说："为义而死的，能回天国"；穆圣说："真回教徒处逆境，常抱乐天知命之念"；老子说："及吾无身，吾有何患？"；佛被哥利王割截身体还说："我成佛，先度你。"他们全知道身体是暂时的躯壳，性灵才是万古长存的。为了借假修真，才肯牺牲肉体，完成大道。

王善人说："身尽情理结人缘，心存道理结神缘，性存天理结佛缘。我守墓到一百天，守灵了三界，诸佛诸祖都来相会，便立志舍身救世化人，请求讲病与学道之人日见增多，才结下众人缘。"

walk the Dao, which in actuality means the great highway of unraveling the mystery of your ancestors and returning to your roots.

Confucius practiced Reciprocity, Jesus practiced Universal Love, Muhammad practiced Magnanimity, Laozi employed the Principle of Stimulus and Response, and the Buddha practiced Empathy. The founders of the five great religions all employed benevolence and walked the Dao of Heaven. They all knew that the Body is but a stinking bag of skin bound to spoil and rot sooner or later, and that only the Heavenly Nature is able to exist for eternity. For this reason, Confucius advocated dying for the sake of practicing Empathy. Jesus stated that those who have died for the sake of Righteousness return to the Kingdom of Heaven. Mohammed asserted that true Muslims must embrace a positive attitude in the face of adversity. Laozi asked, "If I had no body, what would I have to worry about?" And when the Buddha was getting hacked to pieces by King Kalinga in a past lifetime, he still stated: "Before I attain Buddhahood, I must first deliver you to salvation." All of these teachers knew that the Body is nothing but a temporary shell and that only the soul persists till eternity. Borrowing falsehood to cultivate truth, they were willing to sacrifice their flesh and blood and brought the Great Dao to completion.

The venerable Wang Fengyi said: "By fully living out the Ordering Principle of our Emotions (*qingli*), the Body ties us to our karmic destiny as humans. By harboring the Ordering Principle of the Dao (*daoli*), our Heart ties us to our karmic destiny as spirit. By harboring the Ordering Principle of Heaven (*tianli*), our Inner Nature ties us to our karmic destiny as Buddha. I guarded the tomb for 100 days and I guarded my spirit through the Three Realms. When all the ancestors and Buddhas came and gathered together, I made the commitment to dedicate my life to saving the world and changing humanity. The number of people who ask to have their illness explained and want to study the Dao is increasing with each passing day, tying me to the karmic destiny of great numbers of people."

CHAPTER THREE

三界分清

A Clear Distinction Between
the Three Realms

万教都以人为本，性、心、身三界是人的本。哪一界不会，应向哪一界去求。身是应万物的，有不会做的活，要努力去学，越做越有力，越学越精进；心是存万理的，有不会办的事，要向人请教，要专心研究，格物透了就能豁然贯通；性是聚万灵的，要存天理，以天理行事，便和天接灵。

人为什么不灵了呢？因性中有禀性，遮蔽了天性，遇事一耍脾气，天性就混了；心有私欲，遮蔽了良心，恣情纵欲，不怕天理，不顾道理，做些违背人伦、丧天害理的事，物迷心窍就糊涂了；身上要有嗜好，享受不到就生烦恼，享受过度则伤身败德。譬如好赌的，一到赌场就迈不动步，耍起钱来，通宵达旦，腰酸背痛，劳神伤财，事业失败。

The thousands of teachings all take Humanity as their root, and the Three Realms – the Inner Nature, Heart, and Body – in turn are the root of Humanity. Whichever realm you have not mastered, this is the realm that you should pursue. The Body is that aspect of us that responds to the material world. If there are jobs here that you don't know how to do, just study them with earnest effort. The more you do them, the more strength you will have; the more you study them, the more progress you will make. The Heart is that aspect of us that harbors the myriad principles. If there is a matter that you are unable to handle, ask others to teach you, and research it with a focused heart. When you investigate the material world, once you have penetrated it, you will suddenly be able to see everything with great clarity. The Inner Nature is that aspect of us that fuses the myriad aspects of the divine. Harbor the Ordering Principle of Heaven and employ it to handle your affairs, and you will harmonize with Heaven and join with the divine.

Why are we humans not in touch with the Divine? Because within our Inner Nature, there is what is called *bingxing*,[8] our Inherited Nature, which has concealed our Heavenly Nature (*tianxing*). When we run into a problem, we immediately want to throw a fit, and thus our Heavenly Nature gets muddied. In our Heart, there are selfish desires, which cloud over our moral conscience. Letting our emotions rule us and giving free reign to our desires, we do not fear the Ordering Principle of Heaven (*tianli*) nor heed the Ordering Principle of the Dao (*daoli*). As a consequence, we commit acts that violate the rules of human relationships and cause us to lose our beloved connection to Heaven and transgress against its Ordering Principle. Because we are led astray by material things, the Heart becomes confused. At the level of the Body, lastly, we have addictions and cravings. If we do not get to indulge in them, we become annoyed and angry. If we overindulge in them, this injures the Body and corrupts Virtue. People who are addicted to gambling, for example, refuse to move a single step once they enter the gambling hall

---

8 The translation of the term *bingxing* 禀性 has been the subject of many discussions. We have ended up choosing a literal translation, in order to remain true to the original Chinese text. The term as such does not carry a positive or negative connotation, whether in English or in the original Chinese. It is important to note, however, that the specific sense in which Wang Fengyi uses is limited strictly to the negative aspects of what our ancestors have passed down to us, or in other words, the "baggage" that each of us has received from our parents, grandparents, and other ancestors, whether this is directly expressed in their actions or words or unconsciously transmitted through generations.

所以必须以天性为主,才能成己成人。人的天性本来是具足的,只因为身界的不良嗜好牵动心界,心界的私欲牵动性界,才蒙蔽了天性。身界增加不良嗜好,心界就增加私欲;心界增加私欲,性界就增加禀性(怒、恨、怨、恼、烦)。所以必须去习性(吃喝淫赌吸),化禀性,才能圆满天性。认清身子是个物,不能叫物引诱动了心。动了心便生贪求,贪不到手便生烦恼,就动禀性了。所以必须炼得身子动,心不动;心动,性不动,才叫三界分清。

and spend all night until daybreak betting away their money until their backs are sore and their spirit is exhausted, their wealth gone and their fortune in ruin.

For this reason, we must allow our Heavenly Nature to rule us, so that we can mature into our true selves as humans. Originally, our Heavenly Nature is perfect and complete. It is only because our vile addictions from the Realm of the Body lead the Realm of the Heart astray, and because the selfish desires from the Realm of the Heart lead the Realm of the Inner Nature astray, that our Heavenly Nature becomes obscured. When the vile addictions increase in the Realm of the Body, the selfish desires increase in the Realm of the Heart; and when the selfish desires in the Realm of the Heart increase, the Inherited Nature (*bingxing*: anger, hatred, blame, irritation, and annoyance) increases in the Realm of the Inner Nature. Therefore we must discard our Habitual Nature (*xixing*: eating, drinking, licentiousness, gambling, and smoking) and transform our Inherited Nature, in order to be able to express the full potential of our Heavenly Nature (*tianxing*). When we recognize clearly that the Body is just a material thing, it is no longer able to cause other material things to seduce and stir up the Heart. On the other hand, though, as soon as it stirs up the Heart, this generates greed and desires, and unsatisfied greed in turn generates frustration, which stirs up the Inherited Nature. For this reason, we must cultivate ourselves to the point where the Heart is not stirred when the Body is stirred, and the Inner Nature is not stirred when the Heart is stirred. This is what is called "a clear distinction between the Three Realms."

CHAPTER FOUR

清三界

Making the
Three Realms Pure

性界清，没有脾气；心界清，没有私欲；身界清，没有不良嗜好。耍脾气性纲倒，有私欲心纲倒，凌辱人身纲倒，三纲一倒便是恶人。禀性是无始劫来，祖先遗留下来的罪根，人把性化净，没了脾气，才能超拔祖先。私欲是苦根，贪得无厌，苦恼无边，永不满足，日坐愁城。要将私欲去净，才能出苦得乐。不良嗜好是孽根，有嗜好的人，准立不住。譬如好酒的人，一见了酒就想喝，喝得头晕脑胀，乱性伤身。好色的人，见色自迷，贪不到手，心里恼恨，或动杀机，甚至为色杀人，为色丧身，这不都是孽么？人不用死后下地狱，这不是活着就下了地狱么？没有不良嗜好的人，才能敦品立德。

清三界，就是立志用天理捉拿性中的贼（禀性），用道理捉拿心中的贼（私欲），用情理捉拿身上的贼（不良嗜好），三界自然清平。

When the Realm of the Inner Nature is pure, the person has no ill temper. When the Realm of the Heart is pure, the person has no selfish desires. When the Realm of the Body is pure, the person has no vile addictions. Throwing fits of ill temper makes the cornerstone of our Inner Nature collapse; having selfish desires makes the cornerstone of the Heart collapse; and bullying and humiliating others makes the cornerstone of the Body collapse. And when these three cornerstones collapse as one, you become an evil person. Our Inherited Nature is the root of sin that comes to us through eternal cycles of reincarnation, passed down from our ancestors. Only by transforming our Inner Nature and cleansing it until there is no more ill temper are we able to rescue our ancestors. Selfish desires are the root of suffering, resulting in insatiable greed, boundless frustration, eternal dissatisfaction, and worrying day in and day out. Only if you can completely scrub away your selfish desires will you be able to escape from suffering and gain happiness. Vile addictions, lastly, are the root of enslavement because people with addictions are unable to stand firm. Alcoholics, for example, want to drink as soon as they see any alcohol and drink until they are giddy and numb, throwing their Inner Nature into turmoil and injuring their Body. People who love sex lose their mind as soon as they see anything alluring, and if they cannot satisfy their need, they become resentful or get the urge to kill, to the point where they murder somebody or throw away their own life because of sexual passion. Aren't these all forms of enslavement? People don't have to die to descend into hell. Isn't the life of an addict a case of descending into hell while still alive? Only people who are free from vile addictions are able to have a solid moral character and stand firm in their Virtue.

To purify the Three Realms means to make a firm commitment to use the Ordering Principle of Heaven (*tianli*) to catch the thief inside the Inner Nature (i.e., the Inherited Nature, *bingxing*), to use the Ordering Principle of the Dao (*daoli*) to catch the thief inside the Heart (i.e., the selfish desires), and to use the Ordering Principle of the Emotions (*qingli*) to catch the thief that is driving the Body (i.e., the vile addictions). As a result, the Three Realms spontaneously become pure and peaceful.

身界成不怕工作多，能建功立业、身强体壮，是位寿星；心界成不怕事情多，事来则应，事去则静，有领导能力，是位禄星；性界成不怕贬，能容能化，和蔼可亲，有感化力，是位福星。三界一清，福禄寿俱备，哪用向外求呢？

三教圣人，也是从三界修成的道。佛从养性入手，儒从立命着手，道从炼身下手。性中没有禀性，天曹管不着；心里没有私欲，地府管不着；身无不良嗜好，不做坏事，法律管不着。所以人能清三界，就超出三界，直达佛国。

自己吃饭自己饱，自己罪孽自己了。怎么个了法呢？就是要清三界。所以修道要下工夫，绝不是迷信。

In the Realm of the Body, do not fear working hard. Being able to contribute a lot and accomplish great tasks and having a strong healthy body means that the lucky star of longevity is shining on you. In the Realm of the Heart, do not fear having too many matters to deal with. Responding to situations as they come and being calm when they are resolved, and having the capacity to be a leader means that the lucky star of societal success is shining on you. In the Realm of the Inner Nature, do not fear demotion. Tolerance and flexibility, kindness and affability, and having the ability to transform others by example means that the lucky star of happiness is shining on you. When the Three Realms are united in their purity, happiness, societal success, and longevity are all yours. What would there be to search for on the outside then?

The sages of the three great teachings in China[9] also created their Dao on the basis of cultivation in the Three Realms. Buddhism starts from nurturing the Inner Nature (*xing*), Confucianism from fulfilling the Destiny (*ming*), and Daoism from refining the Body (*shen*). When there is no Inherited Nature (*bingxing*, i.e., no negative emotions or our "shadow nature") in your Inner Nature, the officials in heaven will not bother you. When there are no selfish desires in your Heart, the governments of this world will leave you alone. And when the Body has no vile addictions, you will not commit evil deeds, so the laws will leave you alone. Therefore, when people are able to create purity in the Three Realms, they are able to transcend all of them and arrive directly in the land of the Buddha.

When you yourself eat a meal, you yourself feel full. When you yourself commit a sin, you yourself have to deal with it. How do you deal with it? By making the Three Realms pure. In our cultivation of the Dao, we must therefore buckle down and invest a lot of time and effort. This is absolutely not superstitious thinking.

---

9 Confucianism, Daoism, and Buddhism, whose founders are Confucius, Laozi, and the Buddha respectively.

性界清存德，心界清明理，身界清多艺。德能养性，理能养心，艺能养身 - 这是最确实的真理，真行真得，才是真人。

To make the Realm of the Inner Nature pure, harbor Virtue. To make the Realm of the Heart pure, illuminate the Heavenly Principle inside you (*mingli*). To make the Realm of the Body pure, increase your practical skills. Virtue is able to nurture the Inner Nature, the Heavenly Principle is able to nurture the Heart, and practical skills are able to nurture the Body – this is the truest principle in the world. It is only through genuine actions and genuine results that a person can be genuine.

CHAPTER FIVE

三界和三教

The Three Realms and
the Three Teachings

六祖说:"色身是城,眼耳鼻舌是门。外有五门,内有意门。心是地,性是王。王居心地上,性在王在,性去王无;性在身心存,性去身心坏。佛向性中做,莫向身外求。自性迷是众生,自性觉即是佛。"

佛教三皈,皈依佛,是皈依自性成佛;皈依法,是皈依自心弘法;皈依僧,是皈依自身持戒。所以自身持戒得僧宝,心正意诚得法宝,性定生慧得佛宝,戒定慧三位一体,才能普度众生,自明觉性。

道家的三华是:性华开,天理足;心华开,道理足;身华开,情理足。

The Sixth Patriarch[10] stated: "The physical body is a city, and the eyes, ears, nose, and tongue are its gates. On the outside, there are five gates, and on the inside there is the gate of consciousness. The Heart is the Earth and the Inner Nature is the king. The king resides on Earth in the Heart, and when the Inner Nature is present, the king is present, but when the Inner Nature is gone, the king is absent as well. When the Inner Nature is present, the Body and Heart are preserved, but when the Inner Nature is gone, the Body and Heart spoil. The Buddha is made within the Inner Nature, so do not go seeking for it outside yourself. Being at a loss about your Inner Nature is the mark of the masses of sentient beings. Awareness of your Inner Nature is the mark of the Buddha."

In Buddhism, there are the Three Refuges (*san gui*): the Refuge of the Buddha, the Refuge of the Dharma, and the Refuge of the Sangha. The Refuge of the Buddha means to surrender in your Inner Nature and become a Buddha. The Refuge of the Dharma[11] means to surrender in your Heart and spread the Dharma far and wide. The Refuge of the Sangha (i.e., the community of Buddhist practitioners, the monks and nuns and lay followers) means to surrender in your Body and observe the precepts of the sangha. For this reason, when you observe the precepts with your Body, you gain the treasure of the Sangha; when you rectify your Heart with sincere intention, you gain the treasure of the Dharma; and when you make your Inner Nature steady and generate wisdom, you gain the treasure of the Buddha. Only by uniting the trinity of precepts, steadfastness, and wisdom into a single whole can we liberate all sentient beings from suffering and gain self-understanding and awareness of our Inner Nature.

The Three Blossoms of the Daoists are as follows: the Blossom of the Inner Nature, the Blossom of the Heart, and the Blossom of the Body. When the Blossom of the Inner Nature opens, the Ordering Principle of Heaven is fulfilled. When the Blossom of the Heart opens, the Ordering Principle of the Dao is fulfilled. When the Blossom of the Body opens, the Ordering Principle of the emotions is fulfilled.

---

10 A reference to Huineng 惠能, the sixth patriarch in the transmission of Chan Buddhism in China and famous author of the Platform Sutra.

11 Literally "law," this refers to the Buddhist teachings.

儒家的三纲是：君为臣纲得率性，父为子纲得正心，夫为妻纲得修身。

《中庸》上说："唯天下至诚，为能尽其性；能尽其性，则能尽人之性；能尽人之性，则能尽物之性；能尽物之性，则可以赞天地之化育；可以赞天地之化育，则可以与天地参矣。"

譬如人的性是财东，心是经理，身是员工。三界并用，一心一德，才能养性。万德朝宗，万类听命，超出三界，就成道了。

The Three Guidances of the Confucians are as follows: the lord guiding the servant, the father guiding the son, and the husband guiding the wife.[12] By having the lord guide the servant, you obtain an Inner Nature of leadership. By having the father guide the son, you obtain a rectified Heart. By having the husband guide the wife, you obtain a cultivated Body.

It is written in the *Doctrine of the Mean*[13]: "Only those Under Heaven with the utmost sincerity are able to fully develop their Inner Nature. Being able to fully develop their Inner Nature, they are able to fully develop the Inner Nature of others. And being able to fully develop the Inner Nature of others, they are able to fully develop the Inner Nature of things. Being able to fully develop the Inner Nature of things, they are able to assist in the transforming and nurturing activity of Heaven and Earth. Being able to assist in the transforming and nurturing activity of Heaven and Earth, they are thus able to form a trinity with Heaven and Earth!"

As an analogy, we can think of a person's Inner Nature as the proprietor, the Heart as the manager, and the Body as the worker. It is only when the Three Realms work together as a single heart and mind that we are able to nurture our Inner Nature. Consequently, myriad deeds of Virtue will be like streams flowing into the ocean, and myriads of creatures will be complying with their Destiny. When we transcend these Three Realms, the Dao will be brought to completion.

---

12 These traditional Confucian relationships obviously need to be translated from the traditional patriarchal, patrilineal, and strictly hierarchical society of imperial China to our modern times. It is easy to see the lord-servant relationship as equivalent to a modern superior-inferior power relationship in a professional work environment, and to read the father-son hierarchy as parent and child, without losing the original meaning of these power relationships. The husband-wife hierarchy that is frequently referenced in Wang Fengyi's teachings as a manifestation of the natural order of the universe in the human realm, as mirroring the relationship between Heaven (male, yang, husband) and Earth (female, yin, wife) in the macrocosm, is likely to offend modern readers. Because this publication aims to be a faithful translation of the original, and not an interpretation that can easily be applied by the reader, I have chosen to translate the original literally and let the reader make up her or his own mind about what that might mean in our modern culture and in our personal lives.

13 The *Doctrine of the Mean* (*Zhong Yong* 中庸 in Chinese) is a chapter in the Record of Rites (*Li Ji* 礼记) and, on its own, one of the four classics of Confucianism. It is said to have been composed by one of Confucius' disciples.

希望各教信徒，不必是己非人，最好各为己教，信心专一，为人群造福。各行各道、各奉各教。各教都是教人各正性命，如身、意稍有过错，立即用佛教之"忏悔"，基督之"认罪"，孔子之"过则勿惮改"，不可用偏私的心，不可有乖张的性，自然得着佛的妙觉本性，道的真常清静，儒的止于至善。

有人问善人"世上哪个道门好？"善人说"有道就比拉荒（走没有道路的荒地）强。把人当真了是佛，当假了是魔。"

人的所作所为，自性知道，就是天上知道；自心知道，就是地府知道；自己做出来，人人都知道。善人讲的三宝是性、心、身。性是水，心是火，身是土。立身享万物的福，立命享人间的福，立性享天堂的福。

I hope that the followers of each religion do not feel the need to consider themselves right and the others wrong. It is best if they each focus on their own religion and concentrate with all their beliefs on creating blessings for the rest of humankind. Each person shall walk their own Dao, each believe in their own religion. All the major religions teach individuals to rectify their lives, and if they have committed a wrong or made a mistake in their body or mind, to immediately use the Buddhist concept of repentance, the Christian notion of confession, and the Confucian idea that "if you have transgressed, do not fear making changes." You must not employ a Heart that is favoring the self nor have an Inner Nature that is unreasonably demanding. As a result, you will spontaneously achieve the Buddhists' mysterious awareness of the original Inner Nature, the Daoists' constant quietude, and the Confucian goal of reaching utmost goodness.

A person once asked the venerable Wang Fengyi: "Among all the teachings in the world, which Dao is the right one?" He replied: "Having a Dao is always stronger than roaming in an uncharted wasteland. What makes people genuine is the Buddha, what makes people false is a demon."

Whatever it is that people do, if they know it from their Inner Nature, this means that they know it at the level of Heaven; if they know it from their Heart, this means that they know it at the level of Earth; and if they act purely out of their own volition, this is what all humans know. The three treasures that the venerable Wang Fengyi talked about are the Inner Nature, the Heart, and the Body. The Inner Nature is Water, the Heart is Fire, and the Body is Earth. When you firmly establish the Body, you get to enjoy the blessings of the myriad material things. When you firmly establish your Destiny, you get to enjoy the blessings of human-to-human interactions. When you firmly establish your Inner Nature, you get to enjoy the blessings of Heaven.

CHAPTER SIX

三性

The Three Kinds of Human Nature

性是万物的本，所以佛说，一切众生皆含佛性。不过我们人得天独厚，要以天性作事，能聚万灵，为天地人三界的主宰。《三字经》上说："人之初，性本善，性相近，习相远。"这话是不错的。

性有天性、禀性、习性之分。以天性为主的，性情温柔，对人和蔼，爱人以德，看人都好，领人为善；用禀性当人的，总是哭丧着脸，满怀怨恨，看谁都不顺眼，穷凶极恶；有习性的人，见着所好的，如酒色等，就流连忘返，遇见谁，拉谁下水。

有人问善人："孟子讲性善，荀子说性恶，告子说性可善可恶，到底谁讲得对呢？"

The Inner Nature (*xing*) is the root of all things in this world, which is why the Buddha said that all sentient beings have a Buddha Nature. Nevertheless, as humans we are the recipients of a singular generosity from Heaven and if we align our actions with our Heavenly Nature, we are able to fuse the myriad aspects of the divine and serve as the leaders of the Three Realms Heaven, Earth, and Humanity. As the *Three Character Classic*[14] states, "In the beginning of human life, the Inner Nature is originally marked by goodness. By our Nature, we are similar, but our habits make us different." This statement is correct.

The Inner Nature can be differentiated into the Heavenly Nature (*tianxing*), the Inherited Nature (*bingxing*), and the Habitual Nature (*xixing*). If the Heavenly Nature is dominant, such a person's disposition is warm and gentle, and they treat others amiably. They love others with virtue, regard all others as good, and lead others with kindness. If they treat others on the basis of their Inherited Nature, they constantly carry around a long face and are filled with resentment and hatred. They dislike anybody they encounter and act with great viciousness. People who act out of their Habitual Nature, lastly, forget everything around them as soon as they see the object of their desire, such as alcohol or sex, and drag anybody they encounter down with them into the morass of corruption.

Somebody once asked the venerable Wang Fengyi: "Mengzi taught that the Inner Nature is good, Xunzi explained that the Inner Nature is bad, and Gaozi stated that it can be good or it can be bad. In the end, whose teachings are correct?"

---

14 *San Zi Jing* 三字经: A traditional Chinese textbook that is used to teach children about Chinese language and culture in condensed rhythmic phrases of three characters each.

善人说全对！孟子讲性善，是指天性说的，荀子说性恶，是指禀性说的。告子讲性可善可恶，是指习性说的。天性是纯善的，禀性是万恶的，习性是习染的，近朱则赤，近墨则黑。天性流露出来的，是仁义礼智信；禀性表现出来的，是怒恨怨恼烦；习性指的是，吃喝嫖赌吸。习性越多，禀性越大，天性越被蒙蔽。习性累心，增长禀性，遮障天性，失去本性，喧宾夺主，倒行逆施。

习性是孽，禀性是罪，天性是德。习性要善，先去嗜好；禀性要化，先去我见；天性要明，先去私欲。去了习性，化了禀性，圆满了天性，才能行道做德。

Wang Fengyi responded that they are all correct! When Mengzi taught that the Inner Nature is good, he was talking about the Heavenly Nature, and when Xunzi said that the Inner Nature is bad, he was talking about the Inherited Nature. Gaozi's statement that the Inner Nature can be good or bad refers to the Habitual Nature. The Heavenly Nature is pure goodness, while the Inherited Nature is completely bad. The Habitual Nature is contaminated by our habits: It turns red when exposed to vermilion, and black when exposed to soot-based ink. The Heavenly Nature reveals itself as Empathy, Righteousness, Propriety, Wisdom, and Integrity. The Inherited Nature manifests as Anger, Hatred, Blame, Irritation, and Annoyance. And the Habitual Nature points to gluttony, drinking alcohol, prostitution, gambling, and smoking. The more excessive the Habitual Nature is and the stronger the Inherited Nature is, the more the Heavenly Nature is obscured. The Habitual Nature tires out the Heart, causes the Inherited Nature to grow stronger, and hides and obstructs the Heavenly Nature. As our original Nature is lost, the guest overpowers and supersedes the host, perverting our actions and behaviors.

The Habitual Nature is Enslavement, the Inherited Nature is Transgression, and the Heavenly Nature is Virtue. To make the Habitual Nature good, get rid of your addictions. To transform the Inherited Nature, first abandon your self-centered perspective. To make your Heavenly Nature shine, first get rid of your selfish desires. Only after the Habitual Nature is discarded, the Inherited Nature transformed, and the Heavenly Nature fully expressed is it possible to walk the Dao and act in Virtue.

CHAPTER SEVEN

三命

The Three Kinds
of Destiny

命有天命、宿命、阴命。王善人说:"性和天命合,道义就是天命;心和宿命合,智能就是宿命;身和阴命合,禀性就是阴命。把这三个命研究明白,你要用好心,你的命必好。命好命不好,全在乎自己,哪用算命呢?"

命是互相消长的,天命大,宿命必大。宿命大的,做好事就长天命,做坏事就造阴命。宿命小的人,要能抱住本分,尽心竭力,把事作好,众人赞成,便长天命。天命长了,宿命也跟着长。有了宿命,向上尽忠、尽孝,长天命;只养妻子是宿命;吃喝玩乐是造阴命;做事存天理,和天算帐,不与人争论是非短长,长天命;作事心存道理,忠诚尽职,长宿命;没有嗜好,不耍脾气,就不造阴命。天命人吃亏乐,宿命人吃亏不乐,阴命人不占便宜就生气。有天命,掌天权;有宿命,得人权;造阴命,地狱有份。率性当人,长天命;心正作事,长宿命;身成喜欢工作,也长宿命;好逸恶劳、专讲享受造阴命。行道的人,为众人是天命,为家庭是宿命,为自己是阴命。

Human Destiny (*ming*) includes the Heavenly Destiny (*tianming*), the Karmic Destiny (*suming* 宿命), and the Yin Destiny (*yinming* 阴命). The venerable Wang Fengyi explained: "The Inner Nature is linked to the Heavenly Destiny, and Dao and Righteousness are the manifestation of the Heavenly Destiny. The Heart is linked to the Karmic Destiny, and wisdom and skills are the manifestation of the Karmic Destiny. The Body is linked to the Yin Destiny, and the Inherited Nature is the manifestation of the Yin Destiny. Investigate these three kinds of Destiny until you understand them well. Make good use of your Heart, and your Destiny is bound to become good. Whether your Destiny is good or not depends entirely on you alone. So what use is there in going to a fortune teller to calculate your Destiny?"

The three kinds of Destiny wax and wane in relation to each other: When your Heavenly Destiny is large, your Karmic Destiny must also be large. With a large Karmic Destiny, doing good deeds makes your Heavenly Destiny grow, while doing bad deeds builds up your Yin Destiny. People with a small Karmic Destiny must try to firmly embrace that aspect of their self that is originally endowed with the Buddha-nature and put all their heart and soul into their work of doing good deeds so that they are met with approval from the rest of humanity. In this way they can make their Heavenly Destiny grow, and when the Heavenly Destiny has grown, the Karmic Destiny also grows alongside it. For the Karmic Destiny that you do have, spare no efforts in your loyalty to your superiors and in your practice of *xiao*,[15] and thereby you can make your Heavenly Destiny grow. Supporting your wife and raising your children only impacts the realm of Karmic Destiny. Overindulging in food and drink and idle pleasures means building up your Yin Destiny. In all actions, harbor the Ordering Principle of Heaven (*tianli*), settle accounts with Heaven, and do not argue with others over right and wrong or good and bad, and you will make your Heavenly Destiny grow. In all actions, harbor the Ordering Principle of the Dao in your Heart, carry out all your responsibilities and duties with loyalty and sincerity, and you will make your Karmic

---

15 *Xiao* 孝: Following Confucius and myriads of other sages throughout Chinese history, Wang Fengyi often describes this virtue as the cornerstone of his moral teachings. Most often translated as "filial piety" or "family reverence," there is no English word that can express this ancient Chinese concept adequately. It is the reverential attitude of love, deepest gratitude, and respect, and the expression of this attitude in concrete service and dedication, to one's parents, and therefore, by extension, to all elders in one's family and then in society at large.

天命大，和人；宿命大，压人。阴命大，吓人。天命大，使人悦服；宿命大，受人恭维；阴命大，使人畏惧。天命要长不要损，宿命要止不要贪，阴命要了不要造。

Destiny grow. Be without addictions and cravings, do not indulge in fits of ill temper, and you will not build up your Yin Destiny. At the level of the Heavenly Destiny, people respond to the experience of loss with happiness. At the level of the Karmic Destiny, people respond to the experience of loss with unhappiness. And at the level of the Yin Destiny, people get angry when they are unable to profit at the expense of others. With your Heavenly Destiny, you hold the power of Heaven in your palm; with your Karmic Destiny, you gain power in the Human realm; when you build Yin Destiny, there is a place for you in Hell. Accepting the leadership of your Inner Nature in your role as a human being causes the Heavenly Destiny to grow. Handling affairs with a rectified Heart causes the Karmic Destiny to grow. Happily embracing hard labor with your Body likewise causes the Karmic Destiny to grow. A liking for loafing, dislike for hard work, and preoccupation with pleasure build up your Yin Destiny. When people who walk the Dao act in the interest of the rest of the world, this is the Heavenly Destiny; when they act in the interest of the family, this is the Karmic Destiny; and when they act in their own self-interest, this is the Yin Destiny.

People with a large Heavenly Destiny create harmony in their interactions with others; people with a large Karmic Destiny pressure others; and people with a large Yin Destiny terrify others. People with a large Heavenly Destiny cause others to gladly submit to their guidance; people with a large Karmic Destiny receive respect and compliments from others; people with a large Yin Destiny arouse fear and dread in others. Regarding your Heavenly Destiny, you want to make it grow instead of shrinking it; regarding your Karmic Destiny, you want to stop it instead of coveting it; regarding your Yin Destiny, you want to absolutely avoid building it up.

"不知命，无以为君子"；不知人，不能达彼岸。知道对方的好处，是知天命；知道人的功劳，是知宿命；知道人的脾气，是知阴命。知命的人，才是君子。好占便宜的人长阴命，好生怨气的人消宿命，好动性（耍脾气）的人消天命。

天命小得会长，宿命小得会修，阴命大得会了。命小得会长，命大得会守，人有三寸气在，就能自修自造。讲三命为的是"了阴命、止宿命、长天命。"

If you don't know your Destiny, you do not have what it takes to become a noble person." If you don't know others, you will not be able to reach the Other Shore.¹⁶ To know the positive aspects of your opponent is to know the Heavenly Destiny. To know the merits and achievements of others is to know the Karmic Destiny. To know the ill temper of others is to know the Yin Destiny. Only a person who knows his or her Destiny is a noble person. People who like to profit at the expense of others make their Yin Destiny grow; people who like to blame others scatter their Karmic Destiny; people who like to stir up their Inner Nature (having fits of temper) scatter their Heavenly Destiny.

A Heavenly Destiny that is small can be increased; a Karmic Destiny that is small can be cultivated; and a Yin Destiny that is large can be discarded. A Destiny that is small can be increased, and a Destiny that is large can be preserved. As long as we have a single breath left in us, we can cultivate ourselves and build up our Destiny. In discussing how to handle the Three Destinies, we say: "Discard the Yin Destiny, stop the Karmic Destiny, and make the Heavenly Destiny grow."

Notes:
1. Material possessions, technical skills, and education are the Karmic Destiny. Therefore it is said: "With money, you can pay your way out of the Three Realms. But the sins that you cannot pay your way out of, these are hard to escape from."
2. Vile addictions and bad temper are the Yin Destiny.

---

16 *Bi an* 彼岸: Literally meaning the "other shore," this is a technical term from Buddhism where it used as the Chinese translation of the Sanskrit term paramita. It refers to the goal of Buddhist cultivation, or in other words nirvana, after the practitioner has left "this shore" of our cyclic existence (samsara) by crossing over the stream of karma.

CHAPTER EIGHT

三身

The Three Kinds of Body

人身是载道之具、成道之器，极为重要。人要是没有身体，心性就没有房舍。所以修道人用身行道，才能助心聚神，助性聚灵。如果专讲享受，纵欲任性，耗神散灵，就会毁身败德，累心累性，成为罪人。所以说"会用身的超三界，恣情纵欲孽难逃。"人身也可分为三品，就是德身、罪身、孽身。

身体是个胎生物，物与物合，遇着物就愿归为己有。不论任何好东西，一到身上准坏。所以说它是无底深坑，永填不满。不用说吃喝嫖赌吸全爱好，只是吸毒一件，不用几年的工夫，就能把万贯家财吸尽，甚至卖老婆孩子，最后吸海洛因，打吗啡，还犯国法，这不是孽身么？

要是好吃懒做，专想享受，工作不努力，怨天尤人，这样越恨怨，心里越难过，日久必病。有病就是受罪，不只犯罪才是罪人，这是罪身。

The Body is a vehicle for conveying the Dao, a vessel to bring the Dao to completion. This is of utmost importance. If humans did not have a Body, the Heart and Inner Nature would not have a house. For this reason, people who cultivate the Dao must employ their Body to walk the Dao if they want to be able to assist the Heart in fusing together the spirit, and assist the Inner Nature in fusing together the myriad aspects of the divine. But if they focus only on pleasure, stubbornly insist on indulging their every whim, exhaust their spirit and scatter their divinity, they simply destroy the Body and ruin their Virtue. Tiring out their Heart and their Inner Nature, they become criminals. Therefore it is said that, "those who are able to employ their Body transcend the Three Realms, while those who wantonly indulge in their whims have a hard time escaping from Enslavement." The Body can also be subdivided into three aspects: the Virtue Body (*de shen*), the Body of Transgressions (*zui shen*), and the Enslaved Body (*nie shen*).

The Body is a material thing born from a fetus and, as a material thing, is connected to other material things. As soon as it encounters things, it wants to have them for its own benefit. Regardless of how good something may be to begin with, as soon as it reaches the Body, it turns bad. Therefore we say that the Body is a deep bottomless pit that can never be filled. You don't need to be addicted to food, drink, prostitution, gambling, and smoking all at the same time, you only have to inhale the poison of doing drugs a single time. Your addiction doesn't have to go on for many years before the drugs decimate all your family's wealth, to the point where you sell your wife and children, use heroin or morphine, and break the criminal laws of the country. Isn't this precisely the Enslaved Body?

If you are a glutton and a lazy bum who thinks only about pleasure, and you do not exert any effort in your job but blame everybody but yourself, the more hatred and resentment you develop, the sadder and sadder you feel. In due time you will invariably develop an illness. Having an illness is being the victim of a crime, except that in this case the victim of the crime is also the perpetrator of the crime. This is the Body of Transgressions.

人在操作时，一心一意地工作，越做身体越强、精神越足、越有乐趣。不论做什么，要能诚心诚意做三年，事业准有成就。王善人做长工，赚了钱给家中每个人买了五亩田，以后就不在家中工作了，往宣讲堂去讲善书，办女义学，立道德会，都是纯尽义务做公益事业。信仰他的人，当时就有数十万人，他这样立身行道，就是德身了。

身体是物，要听从心的指挥，心还得本着天理，克制人欲，降伏肉身，成为德身。如果身尚未动，心先厌烦，做起事来马马虎虎，做的工作少，损坏的材料多，身子闲，心不闲，思前想后，苦恼身心，必定生病。这叫身累心的罪身。身子有嗜好，争贪不已，不惜身命，专丧良心，闯祸犯法，牵累心性。这是身累心、心累性的孽身。人必须不染孽身、不造罪身、归一德身，才能成己成人。

When people do manual labor and put their heart and soul into their job, the more they work, the stronger their Body gets and the more satisfaction and pleasure they find in it. Regardless of what it is that you do, if you only do it with a sincere heart and mind for three years, your undertaking will certainly be successful. The venerable Wang Fengyi worked as a farm hand until he had earned enough money to buy five *mu*[17] of farmland for each of his family members. Afterwards, he did not work with his family but went out to teach about morality and ethics in lecture halls, set up free schools for women, and found societies for moral cultivation. All of this, he did purely as a charity service to the public, with no financial compensation at all. His followers and believers at the time numbered several hundred thousand people. The way in which he established himself and walked the Dao like this is a perfect example of the Virtue Body.

The Body is a material thing and wants to follow the leadership of the Heart. But for the Body to become a Virtue Body, the Heart must be in alignment with the Ordering Principle of Heaven, restrain the human passions, and subjugate the body of the flesh. If the Body is not active, the Heart grows bored and irritated, and when such a person does start a job, he or she performs it in a careless fashion. The tasks that are accomplished are few but the damages created are numerous. With the Body inactive, the Heart grows restless. Stewing and ruminating endlessly troubles the Body and the Heart, and is bound to cause illness eventually. This is called a "Body of Transgressions, with the Body wearing out the Heart." When the Body suffers from addiction, such people become embroiled in endless fighting and greed, stop cherishing their life, lose their conscience, rush into personal disasters, and break the law. As a result, they implicate the Heart and the Inner Nature. This is the "Enslaved Body, with the Body wearing out the Heart, and the Heart wearing out the Inner Nature." We must not allow ourselves to be contaminated by the Enslaved Body and must not build up the Body of Transgressions, but we must instead return to a state of unity with the Virtue Body. This is the only way to manifest our true selves, to manifest our humanity.

---

17 *Mu* 畝: A Chinese unit of measurement, roughly equivalent to one sixth of an acre.

不争不贪，福禄无边。贪来的有过，争来的有罪，搅来的是孽。

天理是分毫不饶人的，必须修道力行才是。

Without fighting and without greed, boundless blessings of happiness and riches will be ours. But with the arrival of greed come breaches, with the arrival of fighting come transgressions, and the arrival of turmoil means enslavement.

The Ordering Principle of Heaven does not make allowances for one iota of deviations. We must cultivate the Dao with everything we have got. That is the only way.

CHAPTER NINE

横超三界

Directly Transcending
the Three Realms

性是天的分灵，当"率性"行道，正心做德，身体力行。性存仁义礼智信五常之德，心明君臣、父子、夫妇、兄弟、朋友五伦之道，身有士（学）、农、工、商、官五行的职业，才能立身行道（五伦之道），发扬五常之德。德能养性，理能养心，技艺养身。性是良知，心是良能，立身行道成德。人能做到这种地步，名分三界，实为三位一体，便是得一万事毕，超出三界外，不在五行中。心正聚神；性定生慧，聚万灵；身喜勤劳，结缘。这种人象太阳似的，走到哪，亮到哪，人人欢迎，个个景仰，有无穷的快乐，才能享受性天真乐。在世时得不着极乐，死后怎能升到极乐世界呢？我所见过的大德，全是在活着时，以道度人，以德化人，至诚感人，归道时，自知时日，到时向大家告别，说声佛国再见，含笑归空。这是横超三界之不二法门。

The Inner Nature is a duplicate of Heaven's divinity.[18] We must accept the leadership of the Inner Nature as we walk the Dao, act in Virtue with a rectified Heart, and use our body to practice what we learn. It is only when the Inner Nature harbors the Virtue of the Five Constancies (Empathy, Righteousness, Propriety, Wisdom, and Integrity), when the Heart illuminates the Dao of the Five Relationships (ruler to subject, father to son, husband to wife, older brother to younger brother, and friend to friend), and when the five occupations (scholar, farmer, laborer, merchant, and official) exist for the Body to engage in, that a person is able to establish themselves, walk the Dao (the Dao of the Five Relationships), and develop the Virtue of the Five Constancies. Virtue is able to nurture the Inner Nature, the Ordering Principle of the Dao is able to nurture the Heart, and technical skills are able to nurture the Body. With the Inner Nature in a state of innate knowledge and the Heart in a state of innate ability, establish yourself, walk the Dao, and bring Virtue to fruition! If humans are able to achieve such a high level of existence, we may distinguish the Three Realms[19] by name, but in reality the three form a single integrated whole, which is precisely the meaning of "achieve the One, and the myriad affairs are accomplished." Such people have transcended the Three Realms and gone beyond, and no longer exist at the level of the Five Elements. The Heart is rectified and fuses together the spirit; the Inner Nature is stable, generates discernment, and fuses together the myriad aspects of the divine; the Body takes pleasure in hard work and creates strong bonds of karmic affinity. Such people are like the sun, radiating light wherever they go. Welcomed by everybody and admired everywhere, they experience infinite happiness in the true joy of the Heavenly Nature. If you cannot find supreme happiness

---

18 The Chinese term used here, *fen ling* 分灵 ("partial/branch divinity"), refers to a Chinese religious practice of taking statues or images of powerful gods or ancestors from an established temple or main shrine to a subsidiary shrine or one's home, with the assumption that the power of the original deity in the temple will thereby be transferred to the subsidiary location. Once a year, these icons need to be taken back to the original place of residence to renew their power

19 Note that Wang Fengyi's Three Realms are not identical here with the Three Realms of Buddhist doctrine (*trailokya* in Sanskrit), namely Desire, Form, and Formlessness. The title of this chapter carries a strong Buddhist connotation, since this expression is commonly used in this exact wording to refer to the direct access to liberation that is promised in Pure Land Buddhism. Translated literally, it means something like "side-ways or lateral transcendence of the Three Realms" (by directly escaping to the Pure Land paradise), as opposed to the traditional "horizontal" progression that requires sustained effort and gradual ascendance through countless rebirths in order to escape the world of suffering and enter Nirvana.

in this life, how can you ascend to paradise after death? All the examples of Great Virtue that I have encountered looked like this: While alive, they used the Dao to save others and used Virtue to transform others, affecting others with their utmost sincerity. And when it was time to go home to the Dao, they themselves knew the exact moment, took leave from family and friends, promised to meet again in the Land of the Buddha, and returned to the great emptiness with a smile on their face. This is the matchless method for directly transcending the Three Realms.

CHAPTER TEN

五行性

The Five Elements in
the Inner Nature

研究五行性理，为养性成道的要素。

人的肝脏属木，甲为阳木，乙为阴木。阳木性人，仁德、正直、有主意、能忍辱、有担当力。阴木性的人，好抗上、不服人、宁折不屈、好说酸话，做事不许人驳辩，多不孝，一生多难。好生怒气，怒气伤肝，头迷眼花，两臂麻木，四肢无力，胸隔不舒，耳鸣牙痛，中风等病。要想病好，必须拨阴取阳，问主意，以仁德存心，爱人爱物，戒杀。德能养性，行持日久，元性复初。

Studying the Inner Nature and the Ordering Principle of Heaven in relation to the Five Elements is the key to nurturing the Inner Nature and bringing the Dao to fruition.

In the human body, the Liver is associated with Wood. The first of the heavenly stems *jia* 甲 is yang Wood; the second of the heavenly stems *yi* 乙 is yin Wood. People with an Inner Nature of yang Wood are marked by the Virtue of Empathy, are upright and straight, and they have Firmness of Purpose (*zhuyi*). They can endure humiliation and have the ability to shoulder responsibility. People with an Inner Nature of yin Wood love to go against their superiors, do not willingly submit to others, would rather break than give in, love to speak with a sharp tongue, do not yield to others when doing a job but insist on arguing about it, and mostly fail to love and serve their parents with *xiao*. They often experience one trouble after another throughout the course of their lives. They have a tendency to get angry, but anger damages the liver. Hence they suffer from diseases like muddle-headedness and blurred vision, numbness in the upper arms, lack of strength in the limbs, blockage and discomfort in the chest, ringing in the ears, toothaches, and strokes.[20] If you want to cure such conditions, you must tell them to uproot the yin and seek out the yang, and ask them to cultivate Firmness of Purpose (*zhuyi*). Tell them to use the Virtue of Empathy to remain present in their Heart, to love all humans and all creatures, and to abstain from killing. Virtue is able to nurture the Inner Nature, and if they can persist in their actions, over time their original Nature will return to its initial condition.

---

20 Clinical note by Henry McCann: Many of the signs and symptoms given in this chapter follow along a Chinese medical understanding of the internal organs and their associated channels (i.e., channels used in acupuncture theory). The Liver channel starts at the great toe but then ascends to end at the vertex. Along the way it traverses the diaphragm and enters the area of the rib cage. The Liver in Chinese medicine is also linked with the eyes as its sense organ. Since the nature of Wood is to move upwards, an important pathology of Liver is hyperactive upward movement of qi, or upward movement of internal Wind. Therefore, the symptoms here, such as symptoms of the head, eyes, ears, and chest, are all within the normal range of symptoms associated with Liver pathology as seen in Chinese medicine.

Toothache may be caused by an up-stirring of Fire from the Liver. Furthermore, the Large Intestine channel traverses the teeth. The *Yi Xue Ru Men* (Ming Dynasty) links the Liver with the Large Intestine and suggests using the Liver channel for diseases of the Large Intestine channel (肝與大腸相通, 肝病宜疏通大腸, 大腸病與平肝經為主).

心脏属火，丙火为阳火，丁火为阴火。阳火性人，明理、温恭谦让、守礼守分、不争不贪、举止合度。阴火性人急躁、好争理、喜夸张、好虚荣、爱面子、贪而无厌，做事虎头蛇尾。有一分阴火，就多一分遮障，一生多苦。好恨人，恨人伤心，心热心跳，失眠颠狂，暗哑疗疮。要想好病，问明理，拨阴取阳，以礼存心，戒邪淫。礼能养心，行持日久，元神复初。

The heart is associated with Fire. *Bing* 丙 Fire is yang Fire, and *ding* 丁 Fire is yin Fire. People with an Inner Nature of yang Fire are marked by the quality of *mingli* (Illumination of the Heavenly Principle). They are mild-mannered, respectful, modest, and accommodating, observant of ceremony and social distinctions, do not engage in fighting or greedy behavior, and their manner is appropriate for their role in society. People with an Inner Nature of yin Fire are easily irritated, love to fight against the Ordering Principle of Heaven, and are fond of bragging. They are vain, concerned about their image, filled with insatiable greed, and they take care of things with a "tiger's giant head and a snake's tiny tail" (i.e., "in like a lion and out like a lamb"). The more yin Fire they have, the more obstruction and self-delusion they live with. They often experience suffering throughout the course of their lives. They have a tendency to hate others, but hating others damages the heart. Hence they suffer from heat and palpitations in the heart, insomnia and mania, muteness and malignant boils.[21] If you want to cure their illness, ask them to cultivate the quality of *mingli* (Illumination of the Heavenly Principle), to uproot the yin and seek out the yang, to use Ritual and Propriety to remain present in their heart, and abstain from wanton debauchery. Ritual and Propriety are able to nurture the Heart, and if they can persist in their actions, over time their original Spirit will return to its initial condition.

---

21 Clinical note by Henry McCann: The Heart is associated both with the physical location of the Heart as well as a wide range of symptoms associated with the *shen* 神, a term associated with the normal ability to sense, feel, and think. It also is associated with ability to maintain normal states of consciousness and interaction with the world around oneself. Insomnia and various mental disorders are therefore as closely related to the Heart as more obvious symptoms such as palpitations. The tongue (and thus the ability to speak) is the sense organ of the Heart and muteness or problems such as post-stroke aphasia are Heart signs. *Tong Li* HT-5 is an important acupuncture point used classically to treat symptoms of the tongue such as muteness, post-stroke aphasia, or stuttering.

The *Zhi Zhen Yao Da Lun* (*Su Wen* Chapter 74) says that, "all pain sores and itching are subordinate to the Heart (諸痛瘡瘍皆屬於心)." Thus malignant boils are also a sign classically associated with Heart

脾脏属土，戊土为阳土，己土为阴土。阳土性人，信实、忠厚、宽大、能容能化、勤俭朴素、笃行道德。阴土性人固执死板、蠢笨蛮横、心小量窄、疑心特大，一生多累。好怨人、怨人伤脾，膨闷胀饱，腹痛吐泻，虚弱气短，面黄懒惰。要想病好，问信实，拨阴取阳，认因果，戒妄语。信能养气，行持日久，元气复初。

肺脏属金，庚金为阳金，辛金为阴金。阳金性人有义气、擅交际、豪爽活泼、敏捷果断。阴金性人残忍嫉妒、虚伪好辩、巧言令色、笑里藏刀。阴金性人多命薄，好恼人。恼人伤肺，气喘咳嗽，肺病咯血，各种肺经疾病。要想病好，问响亮，拨阴取阳，要有养气，找人好处，戒爱（贪）小，义能养肺，行持日久，元情复初。

The spleen is associated with Earth. *Wu* 戊 Earth is yang Earth, and *ji* 己 Earth is yin Earth. People with an Inner Nature of yang Earth are marked by Integrity and Trust (*xinshi*). They are loyal and sincere, magnanimous, tolerant and flexible, diligent, industrious, and frugal, and earnest in walking the Dao and practicing Virtue. People with an Inner Nature of yin Earth are obstinate and inflexible, stupid and overbearing, shallow and narrow-minded, and exceptionally suspicious. They often experience great strain throughout the course of their lives. They love to blame others, but blaming others damages the spleen. So they suffer from oppressive swelling, distention, and obesity, abdominal pain with vomiting and diarrhea, debilitation and shortness of breath, a yellow facial complexion, and laziness.[22] If you want to cure their illness, ask them to cultivate Integrity and Trust (*xinshi*), to uproot the yin and seek out the yang, to consider the karmic relations of cause and effect (*yinguo*), and to abstain from false speech. Integrity is able to nurture the qi, and if they can persist in their actions, over time their original qi will return to its initial condition.

The lung is associated with Metal. *Geng* 庚 Metal is yang Metal, and *xin* 辛 Metal is yin Metal. People with an Inner Nature of yang Metal have a clear sense of justice, are excellent communicators, and are forthright, lively, nimble, and decisive. People with an Inner Nature of yin Metal are ruthless, jealous, hypocritical, and contentious. With saccharine words and an ingratiating demeanor, they hide knives behind their smiles. People with an Inner Nature of yin Metal often suffer from an unfortunate Destiny. They love to be irritated, but being irritated damages the lung. So they suffer from panting and cough, pulmonary tuberculosis and spitting blood, and the various conditions associated with the lung channel.[23] If you want to cure their illness, ask them

---

22 Clinical note by Henry McCann: In Chinese medicine the Spleen is an organ of digestion and its functions describe what in Western medicine would be assigned to a number of organs, including for example the stomach, pancreas, and small intestine. Digestive complaints are therefore signs of Spleen patterns. The Spleen (and Stomach) are considered the source of Latter Heaven Qi in the body, so when weak a person is prone to fatigue. The disease evil associated with the Spleen is dampness which, when accumulated in the body, gives rise to a sense of distention, swelling, and shortness of breath. It also is associated with a puffy or overweight body

23 Clinical note by Henry McCann: Respiratory problems such as those listed here are associated with the Lung. Other symptoms of the Lung channel include some problems of the skin (the Lung is linked with the skin and hair), and problems of the upper respiratory tract such as the throat and sinuses (e.g., sinus congestion from seasonal allergies). Lung

肾脏属水，壬水是阳水，癸水是阴水。阳水性人有智慧、性柔和、心灵手巧、擅精艺术、肯低矮就下。阴水性人愚鲁、迟钝、遇事退缩、多忧多虑，一生受气。好烦人，烦人伤肾，腰腿酸痛，遗精淋症，虚痨肾亏，疝气淤结等病。要想好病，问柔和，拨阴取阳，认不是生智慧水，戒酒。智能养精，行持日久，元精复初。

to cultivate Radiance of Sound and Light (*xiangliang*), to uproot the yin and seek out the yang. If they want to nurture their qi, they must look for the positive in others and abstain from greed for the lower things in life. Righteousness is able to nurture the lung, and if they can persist in their actions, over time their original emotions will return to their initial condition.

The kidney is associated with Water. *Ren* 壬 Water is yang Water, and *gui* 癸 Water is yin Water. People with an Inner Nature of yang Water are marked by wisdom, a soft and harmonious personality, and a nimble mind and deft hands. They excel at art and are willing to lower themselves to accommodate others. People with an Inner Nature of yin Water are dull-witted and slow, shrink back in the face of difficult jobs, and are full of anxiety and worries, so they experience bullying throughout the course of their lives. They have a tendency to feel annoyed, but being annoyed damages the kidney. So they suffer from soreness in the lower back and legs, nocturnal emissions and strangury, atrophy or impotence, hernias, stasis, and knots, etc.[24] If you want to cure their illness, ask them to cultivate Softness and Harmony (*rouhe*), to uproot the yin and seek out the yang, to admit their wrongdoings and engender wisdom and discernment, the Virtue of Water, and to abstain from consuming alcohol. Wisdom is able to nurture essence, and if they can persist in their actions, over time their original essence will return to its original condition.

---

insufficiency manifests with shortness of breath, fatigue, general dislike of wind or cold, and spontaneous sweating such as frequent clamminess of the hands or the body in general.

24 Clinical note by Henry McCann: The Kidney channel starts on the bottom of the foot and runs up the inside of the leg to the abdomen. An internal branch of the channel penetrates from the perineum to the lumbar spine, Bladder and Kidney. The Kidney is the most yin of the internal organs, and (in addition to the channel penetrating the lumbar spine) as such governs the lower part of the body. This includes musculoskeletal problems of the low back and lower limbs. The Kidney governs the urogenital organs including the reproductive function, and symptoms such as strangury (i.e., painful or abnormal urination) and pain in the urogenital area, impotence, or pain in the lower abdomen (e.g., inguinal hernias) are therefore related to the Kidney.

佛教戒杀，就是孔子讲的仁字。仁是德，德能养性，是阳木。真木性人能立，是德的根，有主意，能忍辱，能受气，不动性（不耍脾气），能立万物。行持久了，自然养足元性。

佛教戒淫，儒家守礼，礼能养心，神足，是阳火。真火性人能明，是神的根，知礼达时，聪明过人，能化万物，行持久了，自然养足元神。

佛教戒妄，儒家讲信，信是万善功德母，长养一切诸善根。信能保气，是阳土。真土性人能容能化，是成道的根，知因果，了循环，能生万物。行持日久，自然积足元气。

佛教戒盗，孟子讲义，大义参天，情理足，是阳金。真金性人果断，是成仙的根。知人好处，有义气，缘大，遇事迎刃而解，能创万物。行持久了，自然积足元情。

The Buddhist precept against killing is precisely the same as the term Empathy (*ren*) that Confucius spoke about. Empathy is Virtue, and Virtue is able to nurture the Inner Nature. This is yang Wood. People with a genuine Inner Nature of Wood are able to stand up straight and grounded. This quality is the root of Virtue. They possess Firmness of Purpose (*zhuyi*), are able to endure humiliation and bullying, do not stir up their Inner Nature (i.e. do not lose their temper), and are thereby able to establish things. Acting like this will over time by itself nurture the original Inner Nature to the point of full return.

The Buddhist precept against debauchery is just like the Confucian notion of observing and guarding Propriety and Ritual (*li*). Propriety is able to nurture the Heart and make the spirit complete. This is yang Fire. People with a genuine Inner Nature of Fire have illumination (*ming*). This quality is the root of the spirit. They know when the time is right for propriety, their intelligence surpasses that of others, and hence they are able to transform things. Acting like will over time by itself nurture the original Spirit to the point of full return.

The Buddhist precept against reckless speech is what the Confucians mean by the term Sincerity (*xin*). Sincerity is the mother of the karmic merits from all acts of goodness, and it nurtures all roots of moral excellence. Sincerity is able to safeguard qi. This is yang Earth. People with a genuine Inner Nature of Earth are tolerant and flexible. This quality is the root of bringing the Dao to completion. They know the karmic workings of cause and effect (*yinguo*), they comprehend the cyclical nature of life, and hence they are able to engender things. Acting like this will over time by itself gather together the original Qi to the point of full return.

The Buddhist precept against stealing is like Mencius' notion of Righteousness (*yi* 义). Great Righteousness connects us to Heaven and makes the Ordering Principle of the Emotions (*qingli*) complete. This is yang Metal. People with a genuine Inner Nature of Metal are decisive. This quality is the root to becoming an immortal. They know the positive aspects of others, and they have a sense of Righteousness and deep karmic bonds with their fellow human beings. When they encounter problems, they solve them readily by "meeting them with the sword." Hence they are able to initiate things. Acting like this will over time by itself gather together the original Emotions to the point of full return.

佛教戒酒，儒家讲智，智能养肾，是阳水。真水性人柔和，是成圣的根。能认不是，认不是生智慧水，能养万物，行持久了，自然积足元精。

要想成佛，得严守戒律，存佛心、说佛话、行佛事，当体成真，就是佛了。要想成仙，五气朝元，得照五行性理，拨阴取阳，实作实行，才能得道。孟子曾说："君子所性，仁义礼智根于心，其生色也，见于面，盎于背，施于四体，四体不言而喻。"

不明道的人，说信道是迷信，做道德哪有迷信呢？全要躬行实践，才能得着。

The Buddhist precept against alcohol is related to what Confucians discuss as Wisdom (*zhi*). Wisdom is able to nurture the kidney and is yang Water. People with a genuine Inner Nature of Water have Softness and Harmony (*rouhe*). This quality is the root of becoming a saint. They are able to acknowledge their wrongdoings, and this ability is what engenders the Water of Wisdom and Discernment and gives them the ability to nurture things. Acting like this will over time by itself gather together the original Essence to the point of full return.

If you want to become a Buddha, you must strictly follow the precepts and rules of behavior and preserve your Buddha heart, speak Buddha words, and practice Buddha deeds, in order to manifest your true self in the present body. In this way, you have become a Buddha. If you want to become an immortal and practice "Five Qi Facing the Source,"[25] you must mirror back the Ordering Principle from the Inner Nature in accordance with the Five Elements, uproot the yin and seek out the yang, and be completely genuine in everything you do. Only in this way can you attain the Dao. Mencius once stated: "The Inner Nature of the noble person is marked by empathy, righteousness, propriety, and wisdom, which are rooted in the Heart. Their outward manifestation appears as a mild harmony in the facial expression, exuberant abundance from the back, and precise and nimble execution in the four limbs."

People who do not understand the Dao say that believing in the Dao is a form of superstition. But how could there be superstition in walking the Dao and acting out Virtue? To achieve success, it is crucial that you walk your talk and stay true to your word.

---

25   *Wu qi chao yuan* 五气朝元: A highly advanced Daoist practice of internal cultivation

CHAPTER ELEVEN

五行性識別法

How to Differentiate
the Five Elements in
the Inner Nature

一个人是什么性，可以从形状、面色、声音、行态（即、形、色、声音、行）几方面来分辨。

木性人，身材细高、双肩高耸；长脸、上宽下窄、瘦而露骨、青筋暴露；走路高压有声；说话的声音，直而短，齿音；生气时，面色青而带杀气。

火性人，身体圆胖，体形丰满，柳肩膀；枣核形脸、上尖中宽、赤红面、肉多横纹、毛发稀疏；行动急速，走路上身摇摆（蛇行）；说话的声音，尖而破，舌音；生气时，面红耳赤。

土性人，五短身材，土性人有三厚：背厚、唇厚、手背厚。平方脸，蒜头鼻子，面色黄；行动，沉重踏实；说话鼻音重；生气时，面色焦黄。

We can look at a number of aspects, namely the body shape, facial expressions, sound of the voice, and behavior, to differentiate what kind of an Inner Nature a person has.

People with an Inner Nature of Wood are thin and tall in stature, with straight shoulders. Their faces are long, wide above and narrow below, lean with their bones revealed, and showing starkly exposed blue veins. Their gait is high-pressure and noisy. The sound of their voice is direct and short and issues from the teeth. When they get angry, their face turns blue-green and assumes a look of ferocity.

People with an Inner Nature of Fire have round and plump bodies, with a full well-padded figure and willow-like drooping shoulders. Their face is shaped like a jujube pit, pointed on top and wide in the middle, and has a crimson hue with lots of horizontal lines in the flesh. The hair on their body and head is sparse. They move with briskness and speed, and they walk with a sway in their upper body (like a snake). Their speech sounds sharp and piercing and issues from the tongue. When they get angry, their face and ears turn red.

People with an Inner Nature of Earth are short of stature and have three areas of the body where they are thickset: they have a stout back, full lips, and stocky backs of the hands. They have a square face with a nose shaped like a garlic bulb and a yellow complexion. Their movements are dignified and steady, and their speech is nasal and heavy. When they get angry, their facial complexion turns sallow.

金性人，身段苗条、单薄；长方形脸、颧骨高。面色白、眉清目秀、唇薄齿白；举止轻佻；说话声音宏亮，唇音；生气时好冷笑，面色煞白。

水性人，体型肥胖；猪肚子形脸，上窄下宽、重下额、面色淡黑。粗眉大眼、毛发深黑；行动迟缓，拖泥带水，坐立时均好倚扶；说话声音，慢长而低，喉音；生气时好哭，面色阴黑。

看人的性，先看形，后看色，便知顺逆。

People with an Inner Nature of Metal have a slender figure and feeble body. They have a rectangular face with high cheekbones. Their face is pale with finely chiseled features, thin lips, and white teeth. Their behavior is capricious and their voice is far-reaching and clear, issuing from the lips. When they get angry, they tend to jeer in contempt, and their face turns ghostly pale.

People with an Inner Nature of Water have a fat body with a face shaped like a pig's belly, narrow above and wide below, a heavy low forehead, and a dull dark complexion. They have bushy eyebrows and large eyes, and very dark hair on the body and head. They move sluggishly, as if dragging themselves through mud and always like to lean back when they sit or stand. Their speech is slow, drawn-out, and low, with the sound coming from the throat. When they get angry, they tend to cry and their facial complexion turns dark and gloomy.

When considering a person's Inner Nature, first look at their body shape and then their facial expressions, to know whether it is in alignment or not.

CHAPTER TWELVE

心界五行

The Five Elements in the Realm of the Heart

人心本是至明的，本性也是至灵的，心生邪念，立即迷惑本性，则昏暗矣。心正神足，光明普照，洞彻十方。

心界的阳木，正直、有良心；阴木性，抗上不服人。心界的阳火，谦虚、明理；阴火，争理、贪名、好高爱好。心界的阳土，诚实、信人、心大意大，能容能化；阴土，多疑、心小量窄、好怨人；心界的阳金，会找人好处，人情圆到；阴金，好分辨、嫉妒心重、好恼人；心界的阳水，清静、平和；阴水、忧虑、好烦人。

Originally, humans have a Heart that is in a state of utter brightness, as well as an Inner Nature that is also in a state of utter divinity. When the Heart engenders morally wrong thinking, this immediately leads the original Inner Nature astray and results in darkness. An upright Heart and fulfilled spirit mean that brightness illuminates everything, penetrating the finest cracks in all directions.

Yang Wood in the Realm of the Heart manifests in uprightness and a pure conscience, while an Inner Nature of yin Wood manifests in resistance towards one's superiors and inability to yield to others. Yang Fire in the Realm of the Heart manifests in humbleness and in the quality of *mingli* (Illumination of the Heavenly Principle), while yin Fire expresses itself as fighting against the Ordering Principle of Heaven, coveting social status, and greediness. Yang Earth in the Realm of the Heart manifests in honesty, trustworthiness, a "Large Heart" and great aspirations, and tolerance and flexibility, while yin Earth manifests in distrust, a "Small Heart" and narrow mind, and a tendency to blame others. Yang Metal in the Realm of the Heart manifests in the ability seek out the positive aspects in others and in satisfying interactions with others, while yin Metal manifests in argumentativeness and separateness, jealousy and brooding, and loving to be irritated. Yang Water in the Realm of the Heart manifests in a calm and composed disposition, while yin Water manifests in fretting and worrying and in a tendency to be annoyed.

心界的阴阳,象太极的阴阳鱼似的,互为消长。心念邪正,立即印在性海脑膜上。愚人以为有秘密,那是自欺的想法。人一动念,自性知道就是天知道,自心知道就是地知道,"诚于中,形于外。""人之视己,如见其肺肝然!"这就是说人人都知道。人心一念之微,天地人三界全知道,所以说,意念一动,浪传十方。况且人存什么心,做什么事,就成为什么性。作善事,就长善性;作恶事,就成恶性。都是自做自受,一点也怨不着别人。明白这个真理,就知道人是自己成全自己升天堂,或自己促使自己下地狱。所以古人说:"与上智之人谈性,与下愚之人谈因果"。把心界五行研究明白,总以阳面应事,自然阳长阴消,就是拨阴取阳。

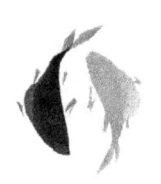

人心就是阴阳关。《金刚经》上说:"发阿耨多罗三藐三菩提心,应如是住,如是降伏其心。"便是上佛国的道。若不自己降伏自己的邪心,就是下地狱的道了。我们能时时注意去掉私心,恢复良心,便能自救救人。才是为天地立心。

The yin and yang in the Heart are just like the paintings of two fish resembling the yin-yang symbol in Chinese art, waxing and waning into each other. The uprightness or wickedness of our thinking immediately imprints itself on our Inner Nature and our brain tissue. Fools believe that this can be kept secret, but that is pure self-deception. As soon as a thought arises in a person, the Inner Nature knowing it means that Heaven knows it, and the Heart knowing it means that Earth knows it. "Honesty in the middle takes shape on the outside." "The way people look at themselves reveals their Lung and their Liver (i.e., their innermost thoughts)." In other words, the whole world knows! The tiniest of thoughts in the human Heart is known completely by the trinity of Heaven, Earth, and Humanity, and we therefore say that as soon as a thought arises, it is transmitted into all directions. Moreover, whatever thoughts people harbor in their Heart, whatever deeds they carry out, these are what their Inner Nature becomes. When they carry out virtuous deeds, they expand their virtuous Nature; when they carry out vicious deeds, they form a vicious Nature. In all cases, we simply reap what we sow, and there is no place or reason at all for blaming others. Once we comprehend this truth, we know that we are the ones who make it possible for ourselves to ascend to Heaven. Otherwise we impel ourselves to descend into hell. The ancients therefore said: "Discuss the Inner Nature with the sages on high, and discuss the doctrine of karmic cause and effect with the fools below." Once you have studied the Five Elements in the Realm of the Heart to the point where you comprehend them, you will always deal with things from their yang aspect. This in itself will cause the yang to wax and the yin to wane, which is precisely the meaning of "uprooting the yin and seeking out the yang."

The human Heart is the doorway to yin and yang. The *Diamond Sutra* explains: "To develop a mind of Perfect Enlightenment, you should thus abide and thus subdue the Heart." This is the path to ascending to the Land of the Buddha. If you do not yourself subdue your own wicked Heart, this is the path to descending into hell. It is only when we are able to constantly pay attention to eradicating our selfish Heart and recovering our virtuous heart that we are able to rescue ourselves and rescue others. Only then do we set our Heart straight for the sake of Heaven and Earth.

CHAPTER THIRTEEN

身界五行

The Five Elements in the Realm of the Body

人的身体是个胎生物，物与物合，容易染上不良嗜好。人心一正，神通性灵，指挥肉身，尽忠、尽孝、发扬人性，光大群性，是君子上达。心邪神迷，一任肉体纵欲享受，毁灭人性，增加禀性，是小人下达。正邪就在一念之间，克念方能致圣。

身界的阳木，端正、能立、建功作德；阴木，身子直硬、傲慢。身界阳火，举止大方、守礼；阴火，拘紧、务外表，做事荒唐。身界的阳土，稳重、实作实行；阴土，拙笨、死板。身界的阳金，活泼、灵敏；阴金，轻狂。身界的阳水，悠闲、儒雅；阴水，懒惰、退缩、邋遢、无力。

Born from a fetus, the human body is a material thing. As such, it is connected to other material things and easily contaminated by harmful addictions and habits. When the human Heart is upright, the Spirit is all-penetrating and the Inner Nature numinous. In command of the Body and the flesh, such a person exhausts the depths of loyalty (*zhong*) and loving service and respect for their parents (*xiao*), thereby uplifting their own Inner Nature and exalting the Inner Nature of all others. This is the meaning of "the noble person attaining a higher level."[26] When the Heart is deviant, the Spirit is confused. Such a person permits the flesh to freely indulge in whatever it pleases, annihilating their Inner Nature and increasing their Inherited Nature (*bingxing*). This is the meaning of "the ignoble person descending to a lower level." Uprightness and deviance are just a single thought apart, and it is only by subduing our thoughts that we may attain sainthood.

Yang Wood in the Realm of the Body manifests in being upright, in the ability to establish oneself, and in grand deeds of karmic merit and virtuous actions, while Yin Wood manifests in a rigid body and in arrogance. Yang Fire in the Realm of the Body manifests in a dignified deportment and observance of the rules of propriety and ritual, while yin Fire manifests in being uptight, in an exaggerated concern for appearances, and in doing things in a flustered manner. Yang Earth in the Realm of the Body manifests in being steadfast and true to oneself in every act; yin Earth manifests in being dull and stubborn. Yang Metal in the Realm of the Body manifests in being lively and perceptive, while yin Metal manifests in being frivolous. Yang Water in the Realm of the Body manifests in composure and elegant refinement, while yin Water manifests in being lazy, timid, sloppy, and lacking strength.

---

26 This is a famous quotation from the *Analects* by Confucius. The second half of this line is found in the following sentence, "the small person descending to a lower level."

人要想成道，身界的行为最要紧。如若放纵，他就无所不为，而且破坏成性。不论有什么好东西，一到身上准坏。身上嗜好一多，能累心下地狱。如能非礼勿动，便可送人上天堂。会用身子，是成道之具、载道之器；不会用，是造孽的机器。没有嗜好的人，心能作主。若是染成嗜好，心就失去主宰能力了。到心中明知不对，可是管不住自己的肉体，人欲来时，就没法自救了。所以必须认清，身子是个胎生物，是幻假不常的，上寿不过三万六千天，叫他累得万劫难逃，实在可惜！所以绝不能叫他做主，只能叫他听命，去立功、立德。

这样把身子降伏住，他才能不为非作歹。释迦佛讲《金刚经》时，王公大臣都执弟子礼，他为什么还托钵入舍卫城乞食呢？就是教育后代弟子不敢叫身子享福染成习性。身上有多大的习性，就是有多大的孽。善人把身子舍了，冻死也不为身体作打算，这才成的道。

For people who want to bring the Dao to fruition, the way in which they conduct themselves in the Realm of the Body is of utmost importance. If they indulge themselves, their actions will know no boundaries and furthermore they will destroy the development of their Inner Nature. Regardless of how good something may be to begin with, as soon as it reaches the Body, it is bound to turn bad. As the addictions of the body increase, they are able to exhaust the Heart and drag it down into hell. But if we are able to not move a finger unless it is in accordance with Propriety, this has the ability to deliver us up to heaven instead. Being able to use the Body means that we treat it as a tool for bringing the Dao to completion, as a vehicle for conveying the Dao. Being unable to use the Body means that it becomes a machine for self-enslavement. In a person without addictions, the Heart is able to serve as the ruler. But if we are contaminated by addictions, the Heart has simply lost its ability to be in charge. Deep in our Heart, we may be keenly aware of something being wrong, but we are unable to control and restrain our body, and when human desires arrive, we have no way of rescuing ourselves from them. Therefore we must recognize that the Body is a material thing born from a fetus, unreal and impermanent, with a life of no more than 36,000 days. Causing it to toil for myriads of eons with hardly a chance to escape is truly deplorable! For this reason, we must not allow it to be in charge under any circumstances but must only make it take orders to engage in acts of karmic merit and Virtue.

Only when we subdue and restrain the Body in this fashion can we prevent it from committing evil. When Buddha Shakyamuni was teaching the *Diamond Sutra*, all the kings, lords, and high ministers treated him with the decorum of disciples towards their master. Then why did he still go out to beg for food in the city of Sravasti? This was to teach later generations of disciples the importance of not allowing the body to indulge in physical comforts and build and contaminate the Habitual Nature. The size of our Habitual Nature is precisely the extent of enslavement we suffer. The venerable Wang Fengyi ceded his Body and did not take it into consideration even in the face of freezing to death. This is the Dao brought to fruition!

CHAPTER FOURTEEN

五行相生

The Five Elements
Engendering Each Other

五行，是用木、火、土、金、水五个字代表来说的。男子法天道运行，是木生火、火生土、土生金、金生水、水生木为顺行。女子法地道运行，以逆为顺，木行水，水行金、金行土、土行火、火行木。

人的内五脏，肝属木、心属火、脾属土、肺属金、肾属水。内五行相生由火起，心属火，心火下降，心中坦坦然，象太阳普照万物，地气上升与天气相合，这是火生土；土的阳气上升为津液，能滋润肺金，是土生金；肺气清，气血变成阳水，阳水是肾水，这是金生水；肾水充满，元精积足，肝气舒畅，是水生木；木得水润，肝气平和，自然心火下降，是木生火。五行圆转，自然百病不生。

The Five Elements are explained by the five representative terms Wood, Fire, Earth, Metal, and Water. Men follow the model of movement in accordance with the Dao of Heaven, which means movement in the direction of the cycle: Wood engenders Fire, Fire engenders Earth, Earth engenders Metal, Metal engenders Water, and Water engenders Wood. Women follow the model of movement in accordance with the Dao of Earth, which means movement against the direction of the cycle: Wood moves into Water, Water moves into Metal, Metal moves into Earth, Earth moves into Fire, and Fire moves into Wood.

Concerning the five internal organs[27] in the human body, the Liver is associated with Wood, the Heart with Fire, the Spleen with Earth, the Lung with Metal, and the Kidney with Water. The internal Five Element cycle of mutual generation begins with Fire. The Heart is associated with Fire, and when heart fire descends, it causes a sense of deep calm in the Heart, like the sun that illuminates all things in the world equally. As the result, the qi of Earth rises and unites with the qi of Heaven. This is Fire engendering Earth. The yang qi of Earth rising and turning into fluids, which are then able to moisten Lung Metal, this is Earth engendering Metal. Lung qi being clear and hence allowing qi and blood to transform into yang Water, which is precisely Kidney Water, this is Metal engendering Water. The brimming fullness of Kidney Water and complete accumulation of the original essence allows Liver qi to course freely. This is Water engendering Wood. When Wood receives moistening from Water, Liver qi becomes calm and harmonious and Heart Fire naturally descends. This is Wood engendering Fire. As the Five Elements move through this cycle, the hundred diseases are naturally prevented from arising.

---

27 This refers only to the five *zang* 脏 organs of Chinese medicine, which are often translated as "viscera" or "storage organs," as opposed to the six *fu* 腑 organs, translated in the medical context as "bowels" or "palace organs."

归到家庭五行，上孝父母是木生火；立身行道，光宗耀祖是火生土；为子孙培德，是土生金；听从母亲的话，殷勤工作，是金生水；母亲爱护长子，是水生木。五行圆转，家道必昌。归到社会上，做事守本分、尽职责，天命必长，是木生火；尊重长上、服从指导，是火生土；立住信用，办事通畅，是土生金；立身行道，培育人才，是金生水；智慧增长，作事胜任愉快，是水生木。五行贪生忘克，则心平气和，五行自然顺行。心性平静，不被事物动摇，才是顶天立地，替天行道的人。

Concerning the Five Elements in the family, to treat one's father and mother in loving service and respect (*xiao*) is Wood engendering Fire. To bring honor to one's ancestors by establishing oneself in society and walking the Dao is Fire engendering Earth. To foster Virtue for the sake of one's children and grandchildren is Earth engendering Metal. To obey the instructions from one's mother and work eagerly and diligently is Metal engendering Water. And a mother's loving care for her eldest son is Water engendering Wood. As the Five Elements move through this cycle, the Dao is bound to prosper in the family. Concerning the Five Elements in society, to be content with one's lot and to fully shoulder all one's responsibilities in handling affairs, as a result of which the heavenly Destiny is bound to grow, this is Wood engendering Fire. To respect one's elders and hence submit to their guidance, this is Fire engendering Earth. To stand firmly and with integrity and therefore handle things with clarity and ease, this is Earth engendering Metal. To establish oneself and walk the Dao and thereby foster talent, this is Metal engendering Water. The fact that growth of wisdom and discernment allows for tasks to be completed with greater proficiency and joy, this is Water engendering Wood. When the Five Elements crave engendering and forget about overpowering each other, the Heart becomes calm and the qi harmonious and the Five Elements naturally move in the direction of the cycle. It is only with a Heart and Inner Nature marked by tranquility and undisturbed by things and affairs that a person can be "holding up Heaven while firmly grounded in Earth" and walk the Dao on behalf of Heaven.

男子若是木性人，有真主意，爱人爱物，做事从容中道，不着急、不上火，这是仁德木，生出明理火，第一步顺运；再能明理达时，虚怀若谷，虚心的人，事情做坏，会反省己过，不去抱怨别人，所以说，"明理不怨人"，能原谅人，信人不疑，这是明理火，生出信实土来，走上第二步顺运；阳土性人，厚道，宽宏大量，遇事能找人好处，有义气，准有人缘，这是信实土生出响亮金来，第三步顺运；金性人义气大，人情圆，遇事做错，自己认不是圆情，认不是生智慧水，这是响亮金生出智慧水来，第四步顺运；水性人有智慧，性柔和，和人合众，博施济众，同情人，爱护人，这是智慧水又生出仁德木来，是第五步顺运。

人走两步顺运主富，三步顺运主贵，四步顺运为贤，五步顺运为圣。

Talking about men, if they have an Inner Nature of Wood, they possess genuine Firmness of Purpose (*zhuyi*) and feel love for others and for all creatures. They handle affairs in an unhurried manner and centered in the Dao, without anxiety and emotional outbursts, as an expression of Wood Empathy and Virtue. As the first step of progression in the direction of the Five Elements cycle, this is Wood giving birth to *mingli* Fire ("Illumination of the Heavenly Principle"). Again, when such a man is able to reach this Illumination of the Heavenly Principle, he will be receptive to others like an open valley and with no preconceptions. If things turn out badly, he will turn around and reflect on his own shortcomings instead of blaming others. Therefore we say, "*Mingli* is to not blame others." The ability of such a man to forgive others and to trust them without a doubt, this is *mingli* Fire giving birth to *xinshi* ("Integrity and Trust") Earth, the second step of progression in the direction of the Five Elements cycle. A man with an Inner Nature of yang Earth is generous and magnanimous. The ability of such a man to seek out the positive aspects in others in the face of difficulties and his spirit of righteousness and strong karmic bonds with others, this is *xinshi* Earth giving birth to *xiangliang* ("Radiance of Sound and Light") Metal, the third step in the progression in the direction of the Five Elements cycle. People with an Inner Nature of Metal have a deep sense of righteousness and enjoy well-rounded relationships with others. When they run into problems and do something wrong, they find satisfaction in admitting their own fault. Admitting one's own fault is engendering the Water of Wisdom. This is *xiangliang* Metal giving birth to the Water of Wisdom, the fourth step in the progression in the direction of the Five Elements cycle. People with an Inner Nature of Water have wisdom and have a Nature marked by Softness and Harmony (*rouhe*). They unite with others to form groups, carry out broad measures of charity work, have Empathy for and take good care for others. This is the Water of Wisdom again giving birth to the Wood of Empathy and Virtue, the fifth step in the progression of the Five Elements according to the cycle of generation.

As people walk two steps in the direction of the cycle, they master material wealth. As they walk three steps, they master nobility. As they walk four steps, they become paragons of virtue. As they walk five steps, they become saints.

女子以男子逆运为顺运。水是木的母，所以木性女子，有真主意，爱人爱物，柔顺待人，有理不争，有错自己认，是率到真水上去了，木得水的滋润，这叫归根认母，是第一步顺运；真水性人，性情柔和，能认不是，有智慧，准能找人的好处，有义气，是水行到金上，第二步顺运；金性人，人情圆，有义气，遇事能委曲求全，宽宏大量，象土地能载万物，承万污，这是行到真土上，是第三步顺运；土性人厚道、宽宏，遇事失败不怨人，不怨人是真明理，自能守礼守分，这是行到真火上，第四步顺运；人能安分守礼，自然不被外物所引诱，才有真主意，这是行到木上，第五步顺运。五行就圆转，内不伤己，外不伤人，是真仁德。

For women, movement in the right direction means to move in the opposite direction from men. Water is the mother of Wood. For this reason, when women with an Inner Nature of Wood, who have a genuine Firmness of Purpose (*zhuyi*) and love others and all creatures, treat others with flexibility and yielding, do not argue when they are in the right, and acknowledge their fault when they are wrong, this means that they have been led upward towards genuine Water and that Wood is receiving moistening by Water. This is called "returning to the root and acknowledging the mother"; it is the first step in the rightful progression of the cycle. When women with a genuine Inner Nature of Water, with a personality marked by Softness and Harmony (*rouhe*), the ability to acknowledge their mistakes, and wisdom, have a clear ability to seek out the positive aspects in others and a sense of righteousness, this is Water moving up into Metal, the second step in the rightful progression of the cycle. When women with an Inner Nature of Metal, who enjoy well-rounded relationships with others and have a sense of righteousness, are able to compromise for the sake of the greater good in the face of problems, have magnanimity and generosity of the mind that resembles the way in which the Earth is able to sustain all things and hold all defilement, this is moving up into genuine Earth, the third step in the rightful progression of the cycle. When women with an Inner Nature of Earth, who are honest and magnanimous, do not blame others when they encounter problems or suffer losses, this is a manifestation of genuine Illumination of the Heavenly Principle (*mingli*). It expresses the ability to observe Propriety and accept one's lot in life. This is moving up into genuine Fire, the fourth step in the rightful progression of the cycle. It is only when people are able to calmly accept their lot and observe Propriety and are naturally not seduced by external things that there can be genuine Firmness of Purpose (*zhuyi*). This is moving up into Wood, the fifth step in the rightful progression of the cycle. When the Five Elements move in a complete cycle, there is no injury to the self on the inside and no injury to others on the outside. This is genuine Empathy and Virtue.

CHAPTER FIFTEEN

五行相克

The Five Elements
Overpowering Each Other

人的天然本性，本来有生无克。一落后天，被气禀所拘、物欲所蔽，就走上克运和逆运。现在研究五行相克。

木克土，土克水，水克火，火克金，金克木。生则发旺，克就受伤。

怎样是木克土呢？阴木性人，自是、不服人，我见太深，更好抗上，又直又硬，出言顶撞，亏孝道。所以说："木克土，不孝祖，先去母。"在本身上讲，阴木性人好动气，土性又死板固执，将怨气闷在心里，脾经受伤，消化不良。所以说"木克土，胃发堵。"对伦常说，轻则把父母克病，重则克死。就是小孩犯木克土，也看得出来，从小就不听父母的话，打死也不肯挪地方。这种性子的小孩，多缺爹少娘，本身也会患胃病。这全是木克土的毛病。要想变克为生，也容易。平素心存孝念，遇事才有主意，不越礼犯分，自然不耍脾气，就明理了。木去生火，便贪生忘克了。要是女子犯木克土，要往水上行，认不是生出智慧水来，便木行水了。

The original state of the Inner Nature in humans is such that there is only engendering and no overpowering. But as soon as we drop into our incarnated state, the Inner Nature becomes constrained by the endowments of qi and obscured by material desires. Hence begins movement in the direction of overpowering and counterflow. In the present section, let us investigate how the Five Elements overpower each other.

Wood overpowers Earth, Earth overpowers Water, Water overpowers Fire, Fire overpowers Metal, and Metal overpowers Wood. The cycle of generation causes us to prosper; the cycle of overpowering causes us to suffer injury.

How is it that Wood overpowers Earth? People with an Inner Nature of yin Wood are self-righteous, do not yield to others, are excessively self-centered, love to resist their superiors, are rigid and inflexible, speak in a confrontational manner, and are inept at the Dao of *xiao* ("Loving Service and Respect for their Parents"). Therefore we say, "When Wood overpowers Earth, such people lack *xiao* towards their ancestors and first get rid of their mother." Speaking specifically about the body, people with an Inner Nature of yin Wood have a tendency to get riled up. In addition, an Inner Nature of Earth makes the person inflexible and obstinate, as a result of which feelings of blame get suppressed and smolder in the Heart. The spleen channel is injured and digestion becomes impaired. Therefore we say, "When Wood overpowers Earth, the stomach develops blockages." In regards to human relationships, in milder cases the parents get overpowered to the point of falling ill, but in serious cases they get overpowered to the point of dying. You can already see situations with small children who commit this offense of Wood overpowering Earth: From a young age, they do not listen to their parents and are unwilling to move an inch even if you were to beat them to death. Children with this kind of Inner Nature often lack adequate parenting and might also suffer from stomach pathologies themselves. These are entirely diseases of Wood overpowering Earth. If you want to transform the dynamic of overpowering to one of engendering, this is actually quite easy. Constantly hold thoughts of *xiao* in your heart; when you run into problems, address them with Firmness of Purpose (*zhuyi*); and do not overstep the rules of Propriety or violate your lot in life. As a result, naturally you will no longer throw fits of temper, which means that you have achieved Illumination of the Heavenly Principle (*mingli*).

怎样叫土克水呢？阴土性人，固执死板，心狭量小，遇事看不开，好生闷气。水土合泥，分不清是非。心里没缝儿，忧虑发烦，脸色黄里透黑，精神萎靡不振，烦人伤肾，亏损元精。对伦常上，少年克母，中年克妻，子女不旺，环境不顺，这是土克水的毛病。若想不克，心里要存家人的好处，遇事不随心，想起平素的好处，就能用大义包涵过去了。这样行久了，生出金来，就走顺运。女子要向火上行，能真明理，自然不烦人了。象阴土被太阳一晒，自然温暖松疏了。

For Wood to engender Water means that it is craving the cycle of engendering and has forgotten about overpowering. In the case of women who commit the offense of Wood overpowering Earth, they must go upward in the direction of Water. Acknowledging their shortcomings gives birth to wisdom and discernment, the qualities of Water, which is precisely Wood moving into Water.

What do we mean by Earth overpowering Water? People with an Inner Nature of yin Earth are obstinate and inflexible, with a narrow mind and "small heart." When they encounter problems, they are unable to accept what they dislike, and they have a tendency to brood in depressed anger. Water mixed with Earth turns into mud, and such people are not able to differentiate clearly between fact and fiction. Having no "seams" in their heart, they worry and become melancholy and irritated. Their facial complexion is yellow with blackness seeping through, and their spirit is listless and depressed. Irritating others injures the kidney and debilitates the original essence. In terms of human relationships, in their youth they overpower their mother, and in middle age they overpower their wife. Their children do not prosper and they are not in alignment with their surroundings. These are the symptoms of Earth overpowering Water. If you want to avoid this dynamic of overpowering, in your Heart you must hold all the positive aspects of your family members, and you must not follow your selfish Heart's desires when encountering problems. By recalling the positive aspects that are ordinarily present, you are able to use Great Righteousness to forgive what is in the past. After you have practiced this for a long time, Metal is born, which means that you are walking in the right direction. When women move up towards Fire, they are able to discover genuine *mingli* (Illumination of the Heavenly Principle) and naturally stop irritating others. This is like shady yin Earth that naturally becomes warm and loose and light as soon as the sun is shining on it.

怎样叫水克火呢？阴水性人，愚鲁不达，心眼慢，欲进又退，还想要好，外表柔和，心里急躁，面色黑红发暗，心经受伤，心神不稳，心热、心跳、患心脏病。在伦常上，幼年克父，女子中年克夫。要想不克，得认不是，时间长了生出智慧水来，遇事就有主意了。水去生木，贪生忘克，就顺过来了。女子要找人好处，水向金上行，就活泼响亮了。

怎样叫火克金呢？阴火性人，又急又躁，好争理，主贪，爱出风头，什么事都有他，好说人短处，就是火去克金，面色白里透红，肺经受伤，容易得肺病，常感冒，咳嗽。家里伤财、克子女。所以说："火克金，爱操心，不丧钱财伤子孙。"要想不克，得学宽宏大量，相信别人，火去生土，就不克了。女子要有主意，不去贪争，生出爱人爱物的心来，火去行木，就不克了。

What do we mean by Water overpowering Fire? People with an Inner Nature of yin Water are foolishly rude and unperceptive, dull-witted, shrink back even though they want to advance, and even when they have the best intentions and are soft and harmonious on the surface, they are irritable and impatient in their Heart. Their facial complexion is blackish red and tarnished. When the Heart channel sustains injury, their mind becomes unstable, and they suffer from heat in the heart, heart palpitations, and heart disease. In terms of human relationships, they overpower the father in their youth, and in middle age women overpower their husband. If you want to avoid this dynamic of overpowering, you must acknowledge your mistakes, and over time the Water of wisdom and discernment will be born, so that you possess Firmness of Purpose (*zhuyi*) when you run into problems. For Water to engender Wood means that it is craving the cycle of engendering and has forgotten about overpowering, or in other words that you are moving in the right direction. When women seek out the positive aspects in others, Water moves up towards Metal, and they become spirited and Radiant in Light and Sound (*xiangliang*).

What do we mean by Fire overpowering Metal? People with an Inner Nature of yin Fire are impatient and at the same time irritable, love to argue over principles, are ruled by greed, and love to be the center of attention. They have to be meddling in every single thing, and love to talk about other people's shortcomings. This is Fire moving in to overcome Metal. Their facial complexion is white with red seeping through, and when the lung channel sustains injury they easily contract illnesses in the lung, like colds and coughs. In the family, they throw their wealth away, and they overpower their children. Therefore we say, "When Fire overpowers Metal, such people love to wear out their Heart with worrying, and if they don't forfeit their wealth, they cause injury to their children and grandchildren." If you want to avoid this dynamic of overpowering, you must study deep magnanimity and trust in others. As Fire moves to engender Earth, it no longer engages in overpowering. When women have Firmness of Purpose (*zhuyi*), they are no longer greedy and argumentative, but give birth to a Heart of loving others and all creatures. As Fire moves into Wood, it no longer engages in overpowering.

怎样是金克木呢？阴金性人，好说人阴私，讦人缺点，暗箭伤人，说话刺激人，自鸣得意。遭人反击，又不服气，内心中分辨不已，来回"拉锯"，就是金去克木。面色青里带白，肝经受伤，肝气不舒，易患肝病。对伦常中人，克弟兄，多灾多难。能认不是，金去生水，自然不克了。女子要往土上行，学宽厚容人，就是金行土了。

如能应克不克，应逆不逆，内则身体健康，外则逢凶化吉，这是人定胜天的妙法。

What does it look like when Metal overpowers Wood? People with an Inner Nature of yin Metal love to divulge other people's dark secrets, expose the shortcomings of others, stab others in the back, provoke others through their speech, and sing their own praises. When they meet with resistance and counterattack from others, they refuse to give in but defend themselves endlessly, responding again and again without being able to let go. This is Metal overpowering Wood. Their facial complexion will be greenish blue with white showing through, and when the liver channel is injured, they suffer from disturbed liver qi flow and easily contract liver diseases. In terms of relationships with others, they overpower their siblings and cause a great number of calamities and disasters. If you are able to acknowledge your wrongs, Metal moves to engender Water and naturally no longer engages in overpowering. When women want to move up into Earth, they must learn how to be generous and tolerant towards others, which is Metal moving into Earth.

If we are able to respond to overpowering movement by not engaging in overpowering ourselves and respond to counterflow movement by not moving counterflow ourselves, internally the body will enjoy radiant health, and externally we will be able to transform any ill fortune that we encounter into good fortune. This is the wondrous method of "human determination overcoming Heaven."

CHAPTER SIXTEEN

五行逆運

The Five Elements Moving Counterflow

五行顺则吉，逆则凶。若是男走女运，女行男运，便是逆运。人是什么性，就有什么命，是丝毫不错的。若想逢凶化吉，就得会率性。所以说应克不克是神，应逆不逆是仙。首先研究五行性，是怎么走逆的？

男子若是阴木性，没有主意，遇事退缩，看什么都不对，心里发烦，这是木逆水，第一步逆运。这种人总是面带愁容，优柔寡断，当做的不做，令人着急，所以木逆水的人克妻。既无能力做事，还不说正经话，遇事分斤拨两，一点亏也不肯吃，便令人看不起他，这是水又逆金，两步逆运。阴金性人，好分辩，疑心大，信不着人，做错了事嫁祸与人。金又逆土，三步逆运。阴土性人，固执死板，又不信人，好往外怨，还自以为不错，愿意叫人说好，这是又逆到火上，四步逆运。阴火性人，好高爱好，又争又贪，不肯安分，瞧不起人，自是心强，目无法纪，心无天理，怒气一生，横眉竖目，凶神一般，杀人放火，毫不畏惧，这是阴火逆到阴木上，五步逆运。一步逆运主贫，两步逆运主贱，三步逆运是鬼，四步逆运是妖，五步逆运是混世魔王。

When the Five Elements move in the proper direction, good fortune results; when they move counterflow, ill fortune results. When men move in the direction of women, or when women move in the direction of men, this means that they are moving counterflow. Whatever Inner Nature people have, this is their Destiny. There is not a shred of doubt about this. But if they want to transform any ill fortune they meet into good fortune, they must be able to lead their Inner Nature. Therefore we say: "To be able to respond to overpowering without yourself engaging in overpowering is to be divine. To respond to counterflow without yourself moving counterflow is to be a saint." Let us first investigate how the Five Element types of Inner Nature can move in a counterflow direction.

When men have an Inner Nature of yin Wood, they lack Firmness of Purpose (*zhuyi*), and they shrink back when they run into problems. If furthermore they perceive everything they look at as wrong and in their Heart they become irritated, this is Wood moving counterflow into Water, the first step in the progression of counterflow movement. This type of a man always carries around an expression of worry on his face, has a weak character and is indecisive, does not do what he is supposed to, and makes others feel anxious. Therefore, a man characterized by Wood moving counterflow into Water is one who overpowers his wife. Now if a man lacks the ability to get things done and furthermore does not speak in straightforward terms, is overly stingy and haggles over every little thing, refuses to accept any amount of loss at all, which causes others to scorn him, this is Water moving counterflow into Metal, the second step in the progression of counterflow movement. A man with an Inner Nature of yin Metal loves to defend his position in arguments, has great suspicion and is unable to trust others, and shifts the blame onto others when he has done something wrong. This means that Metal has moved counterflow into Earth, the third step in the progression of counterflow movement. A man with an Inner Nature of yin Earth is obstinate and inflexible and lacks trust in others, but loves to place blame on the outside. If he furthermore believes himself to be infallible and wishes to make others agree with him, this is moving counterflow into Fire, the fourth step in the progression of counterflow movement. A man with an Inner Nature of yin Fire has a preference for high status and loves high-quality things, is contentious and at the same time greedy, is unwilling to accept his lot in life, and despises others

女子以柔和为本，才能养育万物，要是木性女子，性情刚强，看不起人，又好出风头，好争好贪，嫌男人没用，抢权主事，女夺男位，轻则男人远走他乡，重则把男人克死。所以女子木火性，多守寡，是一步逆运。阴火性女子，说话张狂，不明理，又好挑理，好欺压人，不顺心就怨东怨西，是走到阴土性上了，第二步逆运。阴土性人，不信人，再好说假话，轻狂卖俏，寡廉鲜耻，这是土行金，三步逆运。阴金性女子，好吃懒做，入于下流，为非做歹，走到阴水上，四步逆运。再胆大妄为，天不怕、地不怕，母老虎一般，这是水行木，五步逆运。

while he believes himself to be right, and is strong-willed. With no regard for law and order, with no Ordering Principle of Heaven in his Heart, as soon as he flies into a rage, he scowls fiercely like an evil demon and is ready to kill people or set fire, with not the least bit of fear or hesitation. This is a sign that yin Fire has moved counterflow into yin Wood, the fifth step in the progression of counterflow movement. With the first step in the counterflow progression, the person is ruled by greed; with the second step, by vulgarity; with the third step, he has turned into a ghost; with the fourth step, into a demon; and with the fifth step, into the devil incarnate.

Women must be rooted in Softness and Harmony (*rouhe*) if they are to be able to nurture and rear the ten thousand things. If a woman has an Inner Nature of yin Wood, she is unyielding in her disposition and scornful towards others, loves to be the center of attention, and loves to argue and be greedy. If furthermore she suspects men of being useless, usurps power and takes charge, and forces herself into the man's position, this is Wood moving counterflow into Fire. If this is a minor problem, the man will run far away to another village, but in serious situations she will overpower the man to the point of killing him. For this reason, such women are more likely to be widowed or single. An Inner Nature of Wood Fire is the first step in the progression of counterflow movement. Women with an Inner Nature of yin Fire are flippant and insolent with their words, and lack the quality of *mingli* (Illumination of the Heavenly Principle). If they furthermore love to pick arguments and tyrannize others, and are not in alignment in their Heart but find somebody else to blame wherever they look, this means that they have moved into an Inner Nature of yin Earth, the second step in the progression of counterflow movement. People with an Inner Nature of yin Earth do not trust others. If they furthermore love to speak lies and are extremely frivolous and flirtatious, with no sense of honesty or shame, this is Earth moving into Metal, the third step in the progression of counterflow movement. Women with an Inner Nature of yin Metal are gluttonous and lazy. If they sink even lower and act in wrongful and vicious ways, they move into yin Water, the fourth step in the progression of counterflow movement. And then again, if they act recklessly with great gall, fearing neither Heaven nor Earth, like a mother tiger, this is Water moving into Wood, the fifth step in the progression of counterflow movement.

语云：种瓜得瓜，种豆得豆，心存什么，身做什么，性子也就变成什么样。妖魔鬼怪，圣贤仙佛，全凭自己选择，活着是什么，死后就成什么。可惜人只顾向外去看别人的是非，不知向内省察自己的心性。岂知存什么心，做什么事，就成个什么性。正住心，自然走上光明正道。

As the saying goes, when you plant gourds, you get gourds, and when you plant beans, you get beans. Whatever you harbor in your Heart, and whatever deeds you commit with your Body, this is what your Inner Nature will transform into. Goblin, demon, ghost, or monster, or sage, saint, immortal, or Buddha: the choice is yours entirely. Whatever you live your life like, this is what you will become after you die. What a shame that people are only concerned with looking on the outside at whether other people are right or wrong and don't know to turn inward and critically examine their own Heart and Inner Nature. How could they understand that whatever they harbor in their Heart and whatever actions they commit, this is what their Inner Nature becomes. When uprightness resides in the Heart, you will naturally walk in radiant light on the upright Dao.

CHAPTER SEVENTEEN

五行圓轉

Bringing the Five
Elements Full Circle

五行在运用，运用好了便能超出气数。这是后天返先天的窍妙。全靠自己存心，支配口、眼、耳、鼻、舌不染嗜好，把住自身的贼门。若不从身上入手，一旦染成习性，便连累得意念歪曲。肉体添一分嗜好，心房加一分气禀，便遮蔽一分良知，丧失一分良能。种上烦恼的种子，容易耍脾气。内伤身体，外伤人缘，苦恼无边。若想根绝这种毛病，就得以天性为主，好好运用五行。

五行性的根本是木，木主元性，木性属仁。爱人爱物，敬人明理，明理是阳火。这就是木生火。敬爱人的人，必真诚，真诚是阳土。火又生出土来。土主信实，厚德载物，对人准有义气，大义为金，这是土又生金。仁、礼、信、义，行到圆满，智慧内生，金又生出水来了。仁是统四端，兼万善的。把仁、义、礼、智、信行真，自然五行圆转，不能圆转是由于禀性作祟。阴木性人不服人；阴火性人目中无人；阴土性人有己无人；阴金性人，好捉弄人；阴水性人，讨厌一切人。五行走阴了，怒、恨、怨、恼、烦用事，只知有己，不知有人。一旦得势，不顾双亲。为求新欢，遗弃妻子。对弟兄玩手腕，对朋友打主意。不论任何亲人，不随己意，就生仇恨心，讲报复，动武力，杀害泄愤。所以要想变化气质，必须先去习性。人有身子，就有嗜欲。所以告子说："食色，性也。"不过不可过分。先工作，后享福，抱定忠恕的心，己所不欲，勿施于人，就不至于染上过度的嗜好。君子

Applying the Five Elements well in our daily life can enable us to transcend our fate. This is the ingenious trick to making our acquired state return to its innate Heavenly condition before birth. It depends entirely on what we ourselves harbor in our Heart and how we control our mouth, eyes, ears, nose, and tongue so we do not get soiled by our wants and desires, but guard the gates to our body against thieves. If we don't start at the level of our very own body, as soon as we are contaminated by the habitual nature, we get into even deeper trouble because of the distortion in our thinking. For every fraction of addiction that we add to our physical body, the Heart receives one additional fraction of inherited qi, which in turn obstructs one fraction of our conscience and makes us lose one fraction of our innate goodness. Once we have planted a seed of irritation and frustration, it becomes easy to lose our temper. Internally damaging the body, externally damaging our relations with others, this causes boundless suffering and worries. If you want to exterminate this kind of trouble from the root up, you must allow yourself to be ruled by the Heavenly Nature and apply the Five Elements with utmost dedication.

The root of the Five Element Natures is Wood. Wood rules the original Inner Nature and the Nature of Wood is associated with Empathy. When you love people and all other creatures, respect for others leads to *mingli* (Illumination of the Heavenly Principle), and *mingli* is yang Fire. This is thus a case of Wood engendering Fire. A person who respects and loves others must be genuine and sincere, and genuine sincerity is yang Earth. Fire has thus in turn given birth to Earth. Earth is in charge of Integrity and Trust (*xinshi*), and when your generous virtue carries everything, you will certainly treat others with the qi of righteousness. Great righteousness is Metal, so this is the manifestation of Earth in turn giving birth to Metal. Empathy, Propriety, Integrity, and Righteousness, when these move to make the cycle complete, wisdom is born inside, thus Metal has again given birth to Water. Empathy is what unifies the other four poles, what brings together the myriad manifestations of goodness. When you translate Empathy, Righteousness, Propriety, Wisdom, and Integrity into genuine action, the Five Elements naturally complete a full circle through their movement. The inability to come full circle is the result of adulating the Inherited Nature (*bingxing*). People with an Inner Nature of yin Wood do not yield to others. People with an Inner Nature of yin Fire do not see others. People with an Inner Nature of yin Earth have only themselves

爱财，取之有道。用精神气力换来的钱，用着才心安。例如，有钱的人，想进餐厅，一想父母还没有吃，便买些食物回家，既孝亲又全家享受。由近及远，能孝亲的人，也能爱人。能行"仁"是德，怒气自然不生，阴木性就化了。看见别人的女人，爱慕时，回想一下，假如别人要爱自己的爱人，自己的心里不愿意，即不可胡思乱想，就明理了。明理才能守分，夫妇和，上孝老人，下生贵子，才能享受着家庭的幸福。礼能养心，恨气自然不生，阴火性便化了。遇别人做错事，一想谁不愿意把事做好呢？一定事出有因，就能原谅人，生出信实土。信能养气，不怨人，阴土性就化了。亲友对不住自己，想向他说理，一想人非圣贤，孰能无过，他不仁，我有义，大义包涵，义气大，不恼人，阴金性就化了。自己讨厌别人时，回想必是自己的性子不好，处事哪能全随我意呢？认不是生智慧水，智能养精，烦水自消，阴水性就化了。所以心存伦常道，是化性的无上妙法。自能持其志，勿暴其气。

and nobody else. People with an Inner Nature of yin Metal love to make fun of others; people with an Inner Nature of yin Water loathe everybody else. When the Five Elements move into their yin aspects, anger, hatred, blame, irritation, and annoyance are in the driver's seat, and such people are aware only of themselves, but not of others. As soon as they get the upper hand, they stop looking after their parents. In their pursuit of new pleasures, they discard their wives. They play tricks on their siblings and take advantage of their friends. Regardless of how close they are to the other person, as soon as they don't get what they want, they grow hateful and revengeful, talk about retaliation, resort to force, and murder and kill to vent their anger. For this reason, if you want to transform your disposition, you must begin by getting rid of your Habitual Nature (xixing).

We humans have a body, and hence we have desires and cravings. Therefore Gaozi said: "The desire for food and sex is human Nature."[28] Nevertheless, we must not overemphasize this point. First you work hard, then you enjoy life's many blessings. Hold fast to a Heart of loyalty and forbearance, and do not do onto others what you do not want for yourself. In this way you will not end up being contaminated by excessive wants and desires. The noble person may love wealth but obtains it by following the Dao. Money gained with consciousness and hard work only leads to peace of mind when it is used. For example, a rich man who thinks of going to a restaurant to eat will buy some foods to bring home to his family as soon as he remembers that this parents have not yet eaten. In this way he treats his parents with Loving Service and Respect (xiao) and brings enjoyment to his whole family. Going from what is near to what is more distant, people who are able to treat their parents with Loving Service and Respect are also able to love others. The ability to practice Empathy is Virtue, and naturally prevents anger from being born, and just like this the Inner Nature of yin Wood has been transformed. If you look admiringly at another man's woman but then reflect back for a moment on how you would be upset in your own mind if somebody else loved your own sweetheart, you realize that you cannot indulge in flights of fancy. And

---

28 Gaozi was an ancient philosopher from the Warring States period who is most famous for his discussions with Mencius/Mengzi over the inherent goodness, or lack thereof, of human nature. While Mengzi likened the natural human tendency to goodness to water that naturally flows downhill, Gaozi famously stated that human nature is like wood that needs to be carved into cups or other utensils in order to become useful.

讲五行性，要反躬自问。

木性人问自己有仁德心没有？有我见没有？好不服人不好？看人毛病不看？如果不服人，专看人的缺点，就容易动怒气，怒气就伤肝。火性人自问明理没有？有没有贪、争的心？着不着急？上不上火？为了虚荣、面子着急，上火就要恨人，恨人就伤心。土性人自问，有信实没有？有没有疑心病？度量大不大？量小就好怨人，怨人就伤脾。金性人自问，有义气没有？是不是好分斤拨两地计较？是否好说假话？对人好计较好虚伪，笑在面上，恼在心里，恼人就伤肺。水性人自问，有智慧没有？能否认不是？是否好烦人？烦人就伤肾。

thereby you have gained *mingli* (Illumination of the Heavenly Principle). It is only through *mingli* that we can accept our lot in life, that there is harmony between husband and wife, and that we can treat our elders above us with Loving Service and Respect (*xiao*) and below us give birth to noble children. And only in this way can we enjoy the blessings of our family. Propriety is able to nurture the Heart, which naturally prevents hatred from being born, and just like that the Inner Nature of yin Fire has been transformed. As we encounter a situation where somebody else has made a mistake, as soon as we ask ourselves who would not want to do things right, we realize that there must certainly be a good reason for this situation, and thus we are able to forgive the person. This gives birth to Integrity and Trust (*xinshi*), the quality of Earth. Trust is able to nurture qi, and by not blaming others, an Inner Nature of yin Earth is transformed. When friends or relatives let us down and we are about to argue with them, if at that moment we remind ourselves that nobody is perfect and that while they might not have Empathy we have Righteousness, this Great Righteousness will manifest in forgiveness. When righteousness is great, we are no longer irritated, and an Inner Nature of yin Metal has thus been transformed. At times when we loathe another person, we must reflect back on the fact that it must be our own disposition that is not good and our own desire to handle everything entirely to our own satisfaction. Acknowledging our wrongs engenders Wisdom, the Virtue of Water, and Wisdom is able to nurture essence. As a result, annoyance dissipates naturally and an Inner Nature of yin Water has thereby been transformed. Harboring in our Heart the Dao of human relationships is thus the unsurpassed and ingenious method of transforming the Inner Nature. Being able to firmly hold on to your intention, you will no longer lose your temper.

In discussing the Inner Nature according to the Five Elements, let us turn around and examine ourselves.

If you are a person with an Inner Nature of Wood, ask yourself: Do I have a Heart full of Empathy? Do I have a selfish perspective? Do I have a tendency to not yield to others? Do I look for other people's problems? If you refuse to yield to others and focus on other people's shortcomings, it is easy to have outbursts of anger, and this damages the liver. If you are a person with an Inner Nature of Fire, ask yourself: Do I have Illumination of the Heavenly Principle

常自反省，有毛病，赶快去掉。

认不是生智慧水，找好处生响亮金，不抱屈能生明理火，不后悔能养仁德木，不怨人生出信实土。能时时认自己的不是，处处找别人的好处，不抱屈、不后悔、不怨人，阳长阴消，禀性自然化了。所以善人说"找好处开了天堂路，认不是闭上地狱门。"又说："古人修道，今人不用修，只把性里的五毒 - 怒、恨、怨、恼、烦去掉，就成了。你们听我说翻世界，以为我说大话，其实大事要小办，人是世界的根，人人都能这样翻过来，世界还不自然清平了吗？"

(*mingli*)? Do I have a Heart full of Greed and Contention? Do I feel anxious? Do I easily get inflamed? If you feel anxious and get inflamed because of your vanity and concern for appearances, this causes hatred towards others, and that damages the Heart. If you are a person with an Inner Nature of Earth, ask yourself: Do I have Integrity and Trust? Do I suffer from a suspicious frame of mind? Do I have a broad mind? A narrow mind leads to a tendency to blame others, and that damages the spleen. If you are a person with an Inner Nature of Metal, ask yourself: Do I have Righteousness? Am I overly stingy and do I love to haggle over every last penny? Do I have a tendency to tell lies? If in your behavior towards others you love to haggle and be hypocritical, with a smile on the face but irritation in the Heart, this irritation damages the lung. If you are a person with an Inner Nature of Water, ask yourself: Do I have wisdom? Am I able to acknowledge my wrongs? Do I have a tendency to get annoyed? Getting annoyed damages the kidney.

Constantly examine yourself critically and, when you find any defect, immediately get rid of it.

Acknowledging one's wrongs engenders Wisdom Water, looking for the positive in others engenders *xiangliang* ("Radiance of Sound and Light") Metal, not bearing grudges is able to engender *mingli* ("Illumination of the Heavenly Principle") Fire, an attitude of no regrets is able to nurture Empathy Wood, and not blaming others engenders *xinshi* ("Integrity and Trust") Earth. When we are able to constantly acknowledge our own wrongs, to seek everywhere for the positive in others, to not bear grudges or carry regret or blame others, the yang will grow and the yin vanish, and our Inherited Nature (*bingxing*) will transform all on its own. Therefore the venerable Wang Fengyi said: "Seeking the positive in others opens the road to paradise in Heaven; acknowledging one's wrongs closes the gates to hell on Earth." And furthermore: "The ancients cultivated the Dao. People today do not need to cultivate. They only need to get rid of the Five Poisons in their Inner Nature – anger, hatred, blame, irritation, annoyance – and that's enough. When you hear me speak about turning the world inside out, you may think I am bragging, but in fact great events require small actions, and humans are the root of the world. If all of humanity were able to turn themselves inside out like this, wouldn't the world naturally become pure and peaceful?"

五行圆表

	五元	元性	元神	元气	元情	元精
道教	五方	东	南	中央	西	北
	五阳	甲	丙	戊	庚	壬
	五阴	乙	丁	己	辛	癸
	五行	木	火	土	金	水
儒教	五常	仁	礼	信	义	智
佛教	五戒	杀	淫	妄	盗	酒
	五臓	肝	心	脾	肺	肾
王善人	五毒	怒	恨	怨	恼	烦
	偏性	不服人	争理	欺人	伤人	淹人
	问性	主意	明理	信实	响亮	柔和
	生真	生真木要四样真	生真火要达天时	生真土要认因果	生真金要找好处	生真水要认识不是
	家庭	长子	父	祖父母	儿女媳孙	母

【问性生阳气，消阴毒，聚气凝神，意沉丹田，治病有奇效。】

此表以五脏为中心，五常为物，五毒为阴，用五常之德，养五脏中和之气，去五毒之病根。问性拨阴取阳可以疗病，持五戒养五元可以成道。

138　　TWELVE CHARACTERS

Table of the Five Elements

Daoism		Original Nature	Original Spirit	Original Qi	Original Emotions	Original Essence
	Five Origins					
	Five Directions	East	South	Center	West	North
	Five Yang	*jia*	*bing*	*wu*	*geng*	*ren*
	Five Yin	*yi*	*ding*	*ji*	*xin*	*gui*
	Five Elements	Wood	Fire	Earth	Metal	Water
Confucianism	Five Constancies	Empathy	Propriety	Integrity	Righteousness	Wisdom
Buddhism	Five Precepts	killing	debauchery	reckless speech	stealing	alcohol
Wang Fengyi	Five Organs	Liver	Heart	Spleen	Lung	Kidney
	Five Poisons	Anger	Hatred	Blame	Irritation	Annoyance
	Depraved Inner Nature	failure to yield to others	contentiousness	bullying others	injuring others	flooding others
	Invoked Inner Nature	*zhuyi* (Firmness of Intention)	*mingli* (Illumination of the Heavenly Principle)	*xinshi* (Integrity and Trust)	*xiangliang* (Radiance of Light and Sound)	*rouhe* (Softness and Harmony)
	Engendering the Genuine	To engender genuine Wood, make everything genuine.	To engender genuine Fire, operate on Heaven's time (i.e., make good use of opportunities).	To engender genuine Earth, recognize the Karmic doctrine of cause and effect.	To engender genuine Metal, look for the good in all things.	To engender genuine Water, acknowledge your mistakes.
	Family	oldest son	father	grandparents	other siblings and daughters-in-law	mother

(Examining the Inner Nature generates yang qi and vanishes yin poisons. With the intention deep in the center of your being (specifically, your "cinnabar field"), gather the qi in and "congeal" the spirit. This has extraordinary effects on treating illness.)

In this chart, the Five Organs represent the center, the Five Constancies the material manifestation, and the Five Poisons the yin aspect. Use the Virtue of the Five Constancies to nurture the qi of harmony in the center of the Five Organs and get rid of the roots of illness in the Five Poisons. By examining the Inner Nature and by uprooting the yin and seeking out the yang, we can treat illness; by holding fast to the Five Precepts and nurturing the Five Origins, we can bring the Dao to completion.

CHAPTER EIGHTEEN

家庭五行定位

The Positions of the Five Elements in the Family

在家庭中，祖父母居中央属土位。土主元气。要常提家人的好处是打气，如果老不舍心，好挑剔家人的毛病，便是泄气。父居南方火位，执掌家事，公正无私，循礼守分。家人有不明理的，自己要认不是，怪自己没能教他明理，不怨别人。象太阳似的普照全家。遇到环境不好，要说自己无能，对不起一家老小。若是家长定不住位，一遇失意的事，不是打孩子，就是骂媳妇，火去克金，便伤情了，准有病人。

母亲居北方水位，得承当全家人的不是，免得家人不和，容易出事。

长子居东方木位，得能立，欢喜劳作，赚钱养活全家，并以身作则，家里人有不会做的事，便要怨自己，不可抱屈，抱屈伤心。

其他子女属西方金位，金主元情，心里要存全家人的好处，遇事说好话，化解事端。若是传闲话，就伤感情，主败家。

In the family, the grandparents[29] reside in the position of Earth in the very center. Earth is in charge of Source Qi. By constantly promoting the positive aspects of all family members, the grandparents "pump up" the qi. If our elders, however, are unable to abandon their worries but love to nitpick all the problems and issues of other family members, this means that they are draining qi. The father resides in the position of Fire in the South, wielding control over family affairs with impartiality and selflessness, abiding by the rules of propriety and in keeping with the family's social standing. If there is a family member who lacks *mingli* (Illumination of the Heavenly Principle), the father must acknowledge his own wrongdoing and take personal responsibility that he was unable to teach that person *mingli*, instead of blaming others. Like the sun, his radiance must shine down universally on the entire family. When he encounters external circumstances that are not good, he must explain that he himself is lacking in his abilities and he must apologize to the entire family, young and old. If the head of the household is unable to hold on to his position at the top of the family, as soon as he is faced with a frustrating situation, he will beat his children or yell at his daughter-in-law. This is Fire overcoming Metal and results in hurt emotions and certainly in somebody falling ill.

The mother resides in the position of Water in the North. She must be able to contain any wrongdoings by family members in order to avoid disharmony in the family, which can easily lead to trouble.

The eldest son resides in the position of Wood in the East. He must be able to establish himself in the world, find pleasure in hard work, earn a living to financially support the whole family, and at the same time live in a way that sets an example for the others to follow. If there are matters that family members are unable to do, he must reproach himself but cannot hold grudges, because holding grudges damages the Heart.

The other sons and daughters are associated with the Position of Metal in the West. Metal governs the Original Emotions. In their Hearts, these siblings must hold the positive aspects of all family members, and when faced with a problem, speak positively about it to resolve incidents amicably. If they pass along gossip, this hurts feelings and will destroy families.

---

29 In the context of traditional Chinese society, this refers only to the paternal grandparents.

做家长的主全家的命，如果定不住位，境遇不顺，打骂孩子、媳妇，火去克金，金位人敢怒而不敢言，便抱怨他老大，说："因为你无能，才使我们受气，这日子过不了啦！"金去克木。木位人不肯自己承认立不起来，反怨老人没留下财产，自己累死也没用，向祖父发牢骚，这是木去克土。老人吃不消，怪儿媳妇没生好儿子，没大没小，找起我老人家的毛病来了！土去克水。主妇没处泄愤，便对家长说："看你的死爹，横不讲理，老看不起我们这家人。"水又去克火，必定败家。

家道五行，要怎样才能相生呢？

做家长的人（火位）常向妻子儿女，讲祖先的德性，老人（土位）的好处，是火生土。做祖父母的，不要管事，愿意做就做点，不愿动就领孙子孙女（金位）玩耍，讲故事，教导他们尽孝，告诉他们父母的好处，是土生金。小孩们玩得高兴，做母亲的心里愉快，这是金去生水。主妇精神愉快，便尽心料理家务，注意做活的人（水位）的吃喝一切，是水去生木。做活（工）的人，得到安慰，更加尽心做工，不用家长操心，这是木生火。家里一团和气，家自然就齐了。

The person who is the head of the household is in charge of the Destinies of the entire family, and if he is unable to hold on to his position, and external circumstances are not favorable, he will end up hitting and yelling at his children and daughter-in-law, which is a sign of Fire overcoming Metal. As a result, the people in the position of Metal will develop rage internally but without expressing it outwardly and therefore bear a grudge against the old master, saying: "Because of your inadequacies, we have become the target of your anger outbursts. This life is unbearable!" Metal then goes on to overcome Wood. The person in the position of Wood is unwilling to acknowledge that he himself is unable to establish himself in the world and conversely blames the old master that he failed to leave behind material wealth. Working himself into the ground without any success, he grumbles and complains grouchily about the grandparents, which is Wood overcoming Earth. Unable to bear the suffering, the old grandparents in turn blame the daughter-in-law for her failure to give birth to good children and to take proper care of her elders, thereby causing health problems for them! This is Earth overcoming Water. The mother of the household has no place to vent her anger and hence tells her husband, the head of the household: "Look at your useless father. He is impossible to reason with and he always looks down on our part of the family." Water in turn overcomes Fire, which is absolutely certain to destroy the family.

Looking at the Five Elements in the Dao of the family, how can we make them engender each other?

When the person who is the head of the household (in the position of Fire) constantly speaks of the Virtuous Inner Nature of the family ancestors and of the positive aspects of the elders (in the position of Earth) to his wife and children, this is Fire engendering Earth. When the people in the position of grandparents do not try to take charge of things but involve themselves in minor tasks of their choice and otherwise spend their time guiding the grandchildren (in the position of Metal) in having fun by telling them stories, instructing them in the depths of loving service and respect for their parents, and informing them of the positive aspects of their parents, this is Earth engendering Metal. Small children playing joyfully, bringing happiness to the mother's heart, this is Metal going on to engender Water. When the mother of the household is cheerful in her spirit and puts all her heart into taking care

五行扩充起来无处不是，父母老年（六十岁以上）属冬季居土位，没到冬季，父居火位，母居水位，以在世的祖父母，或去世的先人居土位。兄居木位，弟、妹、嫂嫂等居金位。土位人要如如不动，金位人要会圆情。譬如说：哥哥吩咐做一件事，父亲又叫做另外的事，都要立刻答应，然后酌量哪件事该先做，若是父亲叫做的事应该先做，就要对哥哥说明原委再去做，情就圆了。水位人要能兜不是，对于家中杂物、柴米油盐以及人来人往都要留意，若是出了错，水位人就要兜过来说是怨我呢。木位人主能立，若是家里有不会做的活计，木位人就该说怨我呢。火位人要明理，平素到亲友家去，不是为人情，是为了寻理，和亲友研究办事的道，求明白了，讲给家人听。家里人有不明理的，火位人就应该说怨我呢。这是人人应存的家道五行。

of the household chores, attentively providing all the food and drink for the people who earn a living (in the position of Wood), this is Water going on to engender Wood. When the people who work for a living receive such physical comfort and care, they are able to pour all their heart into their work, and as a result the head of the household does not have to worry. This is Wood engendering Fire. In this way, the entire family gets along harmoniously and the household is in perfect order.

As the Five Elements begin to expand, every aspect is affected. Parents in their old age (above the age of sixty) are associated with winter and reside in the position of Earth. Before they reach their winter season, the father resides in the position of Fire and the mother in the position of Water, placing the ancestral parents, whether alive or passed on, in the position of Earth. The elder brother resides in the position of Wood, and any younger brothers, sisters, sisters-in-law, etc. in the position of Metal. People in the position of Earth should be composed and refined, without being involved in the world, while people in the position of Metal should ensure everybody's emotional satisfaction. For example, if the older brother tells them to do something, and the father instructs them to do something else, with both expecting an immediate response, they must deliberate what task to complete first. If the task that the father is telling them to do should be done first, they must explain the reason to the older brother and then take care of what he asked them to do subsequently, in this way making everybody satisfied. The person in the position of Water must take responsibility for anything that is wrong, paying attention to all the odds and ends in the household, the daily necessities like firewood, rice, oil, and salt, as well as to all the people coming and going. If she has had to expend money, the person in the position of Water must take responsibility and explain that it is her fault. The person in the position of Fire must have Illumination of the Heavenly Principle (*mingli*) and must regularly go to visit friends and relatives in their homes, not to ask favors but to pursue the Ordering Principle of Heaven, to investigate the right way of doing things with friends and relatives. And once he has come to an understanding, he must explain it to the members of his own family. If there are people in his own family who do not have Illumination of the Heavenly Principle, the person in the position of Fire should state that this is his fault. This is how the Five Elements should operate in the Dao of the family for everybody.

父子兄弟地位不同，按照五行来说，父居火位主明理，不论子女怎样不好，只可领教，不可打骂，才算明理。若是子女始终不好，也只能用自责的办法。兄居本位尚仁，弟居金位尚义。不论兄长叫做什么，也不可以有丝毫抱怨才算有义气。如果弟弟不好，哥哥只有怜爱，象父亲对子女那样，才算是仁。老人属土位主安静，不可瞎操心多管闲事。能这样就是性随命转，可说是"率性之谓道"了。

家庭五行方位表

北方水位
（元精）
主妇（母）

西方金位
（元情）
儿、女、
媳、孙等

中央土位
（元气）
祖父母

东方木位
（元性）
领导做工者
（长男）

南方火位
（元神）
家长（父）

The positions of father and son and of older brother and younger brother are not identical. From the perspective of the Five Elements, the father resides in the position of Fire and is in charge of *mingli* (Illumination of the Heavenly Principle). Regardless of where and how a son or daughter may have done wrong, he can only guide them through teaching but cannot hit or yell at them. Nothing else can be considered *mingli*. And even if a son or daughter is acting wrongly from beginning to end, he is still only able to employ the method of self-reproach. The older brother resides in the position of Wood, which values Empathy, while the younger brother resides in the position of Metal, which values Righteousness. Regardless of what the older brother asks the younger brother to do, he must not carry even the slightest hint of resentment, or he cannot be considered righteous. If the younger brother makes a mistake, the older brother must still only embrace him with tender love, like a father towards his children, or he cannot be considered empathetic. Old people are associated with the position of Earth and are in charge of stillness, so they must not worry themselves in vain and meddle in other people's affairs. To be able to live like this means to shift one's Inner Nature in accordance with one's Destiny. We can refer to this as "abiding by the Inner Nature, this can be called the Dao."

Chart of the Positions of the Five Elements in the Family

North: Position of Water
(original essence)
main wife (mother)

West:
Position of Metal
(original emotions)
sons, daughters,
daughters-in-law,
grandchildren

Center:
Position of Earth
(original qi)
grandparents

East:
Position of Wood
(original nature)
leading worker
(oldest son)

South: Position of Fire
(original spirit)
head of the household (father)

CHAPTER NINETEEN

四大界

The Four Great Realms

志、意、心、身四大界，是人的去路。研究明白，选一条光明的大路走，好得到正当的归宿。王善人说："三界是人的来踪，四大界是人的去路。"人要来得明去的白，才不枉在人间走一回。

四大界就是佛国、天堂、苦海、地狱，四大境界。志是佛的根，意是神的根，心是苦的根，身是孽的根。佛、老、耶、儒、回，五大教的教主，全是从志上成的道，是创造世界的圣人。神仙、忠臣、孝子，全是从意上成的，是治理世界的贤人。富贵荣华，尚不知足，还争贪不已，自寻烦恼，是扰乱世界的苦人。损人利己，好逸恶劳，只图享受，不事操作，是破坏世界的罪人。

Commitment (*zhi*), Intention (*yi*), Heart (*xin*), and Body (*shen*), these are the Four Great Realms (*si da jie*), the road that humans walk into the future. Let us investigate them until we understand them clearly, so that we may choose a brightly illuminated highway to walk on and eventually reach our proper and rightful resting place. As the venerable Wang Fengyi said, "The Three Realms are the ancestral footprints that we humans arrive with, and the Four Great Realms are the road we walk into the future." It is only when we as humans understand clearly where we come from and where we are going that this round of walking in the human world will not be along a crooked path.

The Four Great Realms are the Four Planes of Existence: the Land of the Buddha (*foguo*), the Heavenly Paradise (*tiantang*), the Sea of Suffering (*kuhai*), and Hell on Earth (*diyu*). Commitment is the root of Buddhahood, Intention is the root of the Spirit, the Heart is the root of suffering, and the body is the root of enslavement. The founders of the five great world religions – Buddhism, Daoism, Christianity, Confucianism, and Islam – all followed a Dao that was formed entirely at the level of Commitment, and all were saints who were instrumental in the creation of our present world. Spirit immortals, loyal servants, and exemplary models of *xiao* (loving service and respect for their parents), all of these are formed at the level of Intention and all are paragons of virtue who put the world in order. Wealth, nobility, glory, and prosperity, those who suffer from insatiable greed and never know satisfaction, bringing great irritation and vexation onto themselves, these are the sufferers who throw this world into disorder. Those who injure others to benefit themselves, who love leisure and detest hard work, and who only pursue pleasure and never engage in physical labor, these are the criminals who destroy this world.

身界人，有己无人，是己非人。只知吃喝嫖赌，花天酒地，不顾父母妻子，不讲良心道德。他看世人全是坏的，如遇着好人劝他，他不但不听，反而谩骂，花些有用的金钱，造下无边的罪孽，强抢豪夺，横行霸道，杀人放火，不畏国法，好勇斗狠，不惜身命，把世界搅成地狱世界。

心界人，贪得无厌，永不知足，勾心斗角，见利忘义，患得患失，苦恼无边。心里没有一刻安静，不但自寻苦恼，而且把世界也搅乱成为苦海世界。

意界人，爱人如己，喜欢助人，知足常乐，不争不贪，能忍能让，广立善功，是治世的活神仙。这岂不是天堂世界？

People in the Realm of the Body only think about themselves and not about anybody else, consider themselves right and everybody else wrong. They only know of eating, drinking, prostitution, and gambling, dissolutely waste their life away on women and wine, pay no attention to their parents, wife, and children, and do not talk about conscience, the Dao, and Virtue. They regard all other people in the world as bad, and if they encounter a good person who tries to give them wise counsel, not only will they not listen but they will conversely hurl abuses at them. Wasting useful wealth, they fabricate boundless crimes and plant innumerable seeds of evil, seizing things by force and tyrannizing others, killing people and burning things down, with no fear for the laws of the country. With a daredevil attitude they love ruthless combat and do not cherish their own life. So they stir up the whole world and turn it into hell on Earth.

People in the Realm of the Heart suffer from insatiable greed, never ever know when they have enough, lock horns to jockey for position, and forget about righteousness when they see profit. They worry about their personal gains and losses with an anxiety that knows no bounds, and in their heart, there is not a single moment of peace and quiet. They not only bring such great anxiety upon themselves but they throw the whole world into disarray and turn it into a Sea of Suffering.

People in the Realm of Intention love others as they love themselves, take pleasure in helping others, are satisfied with what they have and have an attitude of consistent happiness. They are not contentious or greedy, are able to endure hardships and yield to others, and constantly commit acts of vast karmic merit and kindness. These are living saints who bring peace to the world. How could this not be a world of Heavenly Paradise?

志界人，悲天悯人，只知为人，不知为己。一味行道，不惧艰险。象孔子，困于陈蔡，仍是坦荡自如，弦歌不辍。耶稣被钉十字架，三日复活，仍救世人。释迦佛被歌利王割截肢体，还说："我成佛，先度你。"这全是使志的人。志界人，能容能化，造福人群。以心静为净土，以身清为道场。性定聚万灵，创造佛国世界。

People in the Realm of Commitment bewail the times and pity the state of humanity. They know only how to live for the sake of others but not how to live for their own sake. They single-mindedly walk the Dao, with no fear of hardships or dangers. They are like Confucius, who when trapped between the states of Chen and Cai still continued to sing and play his music with self-possessed composure.[30] Jesus was nailed to the cross and when he arose from the dead after three days, still went on to save humanity. When Sakyamuni Buddha was getting his limbs cut off by King Kalinga, he still stated: "Before I attain Buddhahood, I must first deliver you to salvation." All of these are people who live by Commitment. People in the Realm of Commitment are able to adapt freely to circumstances, and confer great blessings on all of humanity. With serenity in their Hearts, they exist in the Buddhist Pure Land paradise of Sukhavati; with purity in their Bodies, they exist in the cultivation hall for the Dao. Their Inner Nature firmly settled, they gather together the myriad aspects of the divine, and thereby bring about the Land of the Buddha for the world.

---

30 This is a reference to a famous story about Confucius being trapped between two states at war. Unable to escape the situation, Confucius and his disciples went for several days with no food and drink, suffering great physical hardships, until they were rescued by an escort from a third state.

善人说：" 用身界当人的，不论做到什么地步，也是个糟心人。用心当人的，不论怎样有能力，也是个操心人。用意当人的，不论事情怎么多，也是净心人，就是活神仙。用志当人的，不论遇怎样逆境，也不动性（耍脾气）是无心人，就成了一尊佛。所以我说，志界人没说，是无心人；意界人知足常乐，是净心人；心界人好争理，是操心人；身界人好生气，是糟心人。糟心人是鬼，操心人是人，净心人是神，无心人是佛。"

身界人，好管人，管人互相结仇，是地狱。心界人，好怨人，心里过不去，天天苦苦恼恼的。所以说，怨人是苦海。意界人，好助人，知足常乐，乐能聚神。志界人，好成全人，认为是应该做的，没有人我的分别，没说的（怎的都好）就是佛。

The Venerable Wang Fengyi said: "When we use the Realm of the Body to engage as humans, regardless of what situations we achieve, we will always be a person with a rotten Heart. When we use the Realm of the Heart to engage as humans, regardless of what competencies we develop, we will always be a person with a preoccupied Heart. When we use the Realm of Intention to engage as humans, regardless of how much work we have to get done, we will always be a person with a clean Heart, which is precisely a living saint. When we use the Realm of Commitment to engage as humans, regardless of what adversities we are confronted with, they will not stir up our Inner Nature (cause us to lose our temper). This is a "person with no heart,"[31] or in other words somebody who has become a venerable Buddha. Therefore I say: "People in the Realm of Commitment have nothing to say; they are 'people with no heart'. People in the Realm of Intention know satisfaction and constant happiness; they are people with a clean Heart. People in the Realm of the Heart love to argue over reason; they are people with a preoccupied Heart. People in the Realm of the Body love to lose their temper; they are people with a rotten Heart. People with a rotten Heart are ghosts, people with a preoccupied Heart are humans, people with a clean Heart are spirits, and people with no Heart are Buddhas."

People in the Realm of the Body love to order others around, but ordering others around causes mutual hostility. This is hell on Earth. People in the Realm of the Heart love to blame others, cannot let things go in their Heart, and are worried and anxious day in and day out. For this reason we say that blaming others is the Sea of Suffering. People in the Realm of Intention love to help others and know satisfaction and constant happiness, which attracts all the spirits to gather together. People in the Realm of Commitment love to perfect themselves and accept this as what they should be doing. There is no more distinction between "myself" and "other." With no need to say anything further, they are simply Buddhas.

---

31 *Wu xin ren* 无心人: This is a Buddhist expression referring to an enlightened being in whom all mental activity has ceased, pronounced *mushin* in Japanese and most commonly translated as "no mind." It has nothing at all to do with the negative connotations of the common English term "heartless" but is related to the Buddhist conception of the heart-mind as the seat of the senses, rationality, ego-consciousness, and feelings, which continuously respond to the material realm we live in. Liberation from this continuous activity of responding to the outside world brings true freedom and peace.

这四大界,是人生的四条去路。用哪个字当人,就作哪种事,便走上哪条路。以身子为主当人的,便走向地狱的路;用心当人的,是走向苦海的路;以意当人的,是走向天堂的路;用志当人的,是走向佛国的路。你用哪字当人,便知道自己将来的归宿是何处了。

These four Great Realms are the four paths that we can walk into the future over the course of our life. Depending on which of these Realms we base our life on, this is the kind of action we take and this is the road that we walk on into the future. If we put the Body in charge of our life, we are walking on the road towards Hell on Earth. If we put the Heart in charge of our life, we are walking on the road towards the Sea of Suffering. If we put Intention in charge of our life, we are walking on the road towards the Heavenly Paradise. If, lastly, we put Commitment in charge of our life, we are walking on the road towards the Land of the Buddha. Whichever Realm you choose to put in charge of your life, you thereby know where your final resting place will be in the future.

CHAPTER TWENTY

一串之道

The Dao in a Single String of Beads

讲三界是为了知道人性的来源。人有天性，才能得天道。讲三界分清，为的是身不累心，心不累性，天性自然复初。讲清三界，为了性清没有脾气；心清没有私欲；身清没有嗜好；去习性、化禀性、圆满天性。讲五行先讲木性，因为木主元性，也是为的元性复初，恢复本来面目的仁德。讲四大界定位，为的是定在志界，志通佛国。志是道的根，性是道的体，忠恕、博爱、慈悲，是道的用，圣、贤、仙、佛是道的果。

简单说，这十二字，全是为了发扬人性、圆满天性、发扬群性、达成天德。德能养性，性定聚灵，灵光充满是圣。道德会的人常说："孔夫子的道，是一以贯之。王善人的道，是一大串子。""一大串"就是指的这十二字。这十二个字所研究的，只是一个性字。人若成道补天地的正气，就是天地生人，人生天地。所以道是天道，这就是性天大道。

We have discussed the Three Realms so that we can understand the source that our Inner Nature as humans comes from. It is only because we humans have a Heavenly Nature that we are able to attain the Dao of Heaven. We have discussed the clear distinctions between the Three Realms so that we can prevent the Body from implicating the Heart, and the Heart from implicating the Inner Nature, as a result of which the Heavenly Nature can naturally recover its initial state. We have discussed purifying the Three Realms, because when the Inner Nature is pure, there is no bad temper; when the Heart is pure, there are no selfish desires; and when the Body is pure, there are no addictions and bad habits. Discard the Habitual Nature, transform the Inherited Nature, and express the Heavenly Nature to its fullest potential. In the discussion of the Five Elements, we have discussed the Inner Nature of Wood first because Wood is in charge of the original Nature, and because it is by restoring the initial state of the original Nature that we recover the true color of the Virtue of Empathy. We have discussed the position of the Four Great Realms because when we are firmly settled in the Realm of Commitment, this Commitment links us to the Land of the Buddha. Commitment is the root of the Dao; the Inner Nature is the human manifestation of the Dao; loyalty and forbearance, universal love, and mercy are the application of the Dao; sagehood, sainthood, immortality, and Buddhahood are the fruits of the Dao.

In simple terms, the twelve terms discussed in this book are entirely for the sake of exalting the human Nature, expressing the Heavenly Nature to its fullest potential, developing the Inner Nature of the masses, and attaining Heavenly Virtue. Virtue is able to nurture the Inner Nature, the Inner Nature settles and gathers the divine, and a person permeated with the radiance of the divine is a saint. People in Societies for the Promotion of Virtue[32] often say: "The Dao of Confucius is the One that threads it all together. The Dao of Wang Fengyi is one large string of beads." This "one large string of beads" refers directly to these twelve terms. What these twelve terms are investigating is nothing but the single term "Inner Nature" (*xing* 性). If people bring the Dao to fruition and thereby supplement the righteous qi of Heaven and Earth, this is the direct meaning of "Heaven and Earth give birth to Humankind,

---

32 *Daodehui* 道德會: These are private associations of members who gather for educational purposes to promote virtue in society on the basis of Confucianism, Buddhism, and Daoism.

婴儿降生以后，听他的哭声就知道他是什么性？哭声急的是火，慢的是水，时哭时止的是土，大声哭、突然停住是木，哭声响亮连续不断的是金性。认清他们的禀性以后，就要按照五行相生的顺序去教他，若是男孩儿是木性，就要常呼明理（火），这是木生火。若是女孩儿是木性就要常呼柔和（水），这是木向水上行是女子的顺运。日子久性就化了，这是教性。稍大一点就会说话，便要教叫他爸爸、妈妈、哥哥、姊姊等，使他知道长幼尊卑，这是教命。常这样做就能正他的性命。

and Humankind gives birth to Heaven and Earth." For this reason, the Dao is the Heavenly Dao, which is precisely the Great Dao of the Inner Nature and Heaven.

After babies descend into this world, you can know what kind of an Inner Nature they have by listening to the sound of their crying. When the sound of their crying is urgent and anxious, this means Fire. When the sound is slow, it means Water. When the crying stops intermittently, this is Earth. Loud crying that suddenly stops is Wood, and crying with an uninterrupted loud and clear sound means an Inner Nature of Metal. After you see through their Inherited Nature, you want to start instructing them in accordance with the order of Mutual Engendering among the Five Elements. If you have a male child who has an Inner Nature of Wood, you want to constantly invoke *mingli* ("Illumination of the Heavenly Principle," i.e. Fire), which is Wood engendering Fire. If you have a female child who has an Inner Nature of Wood, you want to constantly invoke *rouhe* ("Softness and Harmony," i.e. Water), which is Wood moving into Water, the proper sequence of movement for women. As the Inner Nature is transformed in this way over time, this is the meaning of "instruction on the Inner Nature." Speaking in slightly larger terms, you also want to teach them how to address their father, mother, older brother, older sister, etc. so that they understand about young and old and respect and humility. This is the meaning of "instruction on the Destiny." By constantly acting in this way, you are able to make the baby's Inner Nature and Destiny righteous.

APPENDIX OF KEY TERMS

Pinyin ▪ Chinese ▪ English

bingxing 禀性 Inherited Nature: The aspect of our human nature that is associated with the Realm of the Body and the emotions of Anger, Hatred, Blame, Irritation, and Annoyance.

dao 道 Dao: Literally, "The Way."

daoli 道理 Guidance from the Dao: One of the three kinds of Guidance.

de 德 Virtue: The outward manifestation of a person's ability to follow the Dao in their actions, hence also the power that stems from virtuous actions.

deshen 德身 Virtue Body: One of the three aspects of the Body.

di 地 Earth: As in the compound *tiandi* (Heaven and Earth), where it is associated with yin while Heaven is associated with yang.

fan 煩 Annoyance: One of the Five Poisons, associated with Water and the Kidney.

hen 恨 Hatred: One of the Five Poisons, associated with Fire and the Heart.

huo 火 Fire: One of the Five Elements or "dynamic movements."

jin 金 Metal: One of the Five Elements or "dynamic movements."

li 理 [Moral] Guidance: As in the compounds *tianli*, *daoli*, and *qingli* ("Guidance from Heaven, the Dao, and the Emotions, respectively. From its basic meaning of veins in jade, this character has come to mean "texture," "principle," "rule," or even "reason."

li 禮 Propriety: Also often translated as "ritual" or "politeness," this is one of the Five Virtues, associated with Fire and the Heart.

mingli 明理 Illumination of the Heavenly Principle: The manifestation of Virtue that is associated with Fire and the Heart.

ming 命 Destiny: Literally a "mandate" or "order," as in *tian ming*, the "Mandate from Heaven." The Wang Fengyi system differentiates between Heavenly Destiny (tianming), Karmic Destiny (suming), and Yin Destiny (yinming).

mu 木 Wood: One of the Five Elements or "dynamic movements."

nieshen 孽身 Enslaved Body: One of the three aspects of the Body.

nao 惱 Irritation: One of the Five Poisons, associated with Metal and the Lung.

nu 怒 Anger: One of the Five Poisons, associated with Wood and the Liver.

qingli 情理 Guidance from the Emotions: One of the three kinds of Guidance.

ren 仁 Empathy: One of the Five Virtues, associated with Wood and the Liver.

rouhe 柔和 Softness and Harmony: The manifestation of Virtue associated with Water and the Kidney.

san gui 三皈 Three Refuges: a technical term from Buddhism, referring to the Buddha, the Dharma, and the Sangha.

san jie 三界 Three Realms (of the Inner Nature, Heart, and Body).

shen 身 Body: One of the Three Realms and at the same time one of the Four Great Realms, in which context it is also known as the level of the Hungry Ghosts or the realm of physical addictions. The Body is further subdivided into the Virtue Body (*deshen*), the Body of Transgressions (*zuishen*), and the Enslaved Body (*nieshen*).

shui 水 Water: One of the Five Elements or "dynamic movements."

si da jie 四大界 Four Great Realms: Commitment, Intention, Heart, and Body, associated with the Land of the Buddha (*foguo* 佛國), Heavenly Paradise (*tiantang* 天堂), Sea of Suffering (*kuhai* 苦海), and Hell on Earth (*diyu* 地獄) respectively.

suming 宿命 Karmic Destiny: One of the three types of Destiny, associated with the Heart and manifesting in wisdom and skills.

tian 天 Heaven.

tian di ren san jie 天地人三界 Three Realms of Heaven, Earth, and Humanity.

tianli 天理 Guidance from Heaven: One of the three kinds of Guidance.

tianming 天命 Heavenly Destiny: One of the three types of Destiny, associated with Heaven and manifesting in Dao and in Righteousness.

tianxing 天性 Heavenly Nature: The aspect of our human nature that is associated with our true Inner Nature.

tu 土 Earth: One of the Five Elements or "dynamic movements."

wu chang 五常 Five Constancies: Also known as the Five Virtues, they consist of Empathy (*ren*), Righteousness (*yi*), Propriety (*li*), Wisdom (*zhi*), and Integrity (*xin*), associated with Liver-Wood, Lung-Metal, Heart-Fire, Kidney-Water, and Spleen-Earth, respectively.

wu du 五毒 Five Poisons: Anger, Hatred, Blame, Irritation, Annoyance.

wu xing 五行 Five Elements (or "dynamic movements"): Wood, Fire, Earth, Metal, and Water.

wu zang 五臟 Five Organs

xiangliang 響亮 Radiance of Sound and Light: The manifestation of Virtue associated with Metal and the Lung.

xiao 孝 Xiao: Often translated inadequately as "filial piety," this virtue is the foundation of the Confucian family structure and moral value system. It means the loving service and respect for one's parents and therefore by extension of all elders in society.

xixing 習性 Habitual Nature: The aspect of our human nature that is associated with the Realm of the Heart and the bad habits of eating, drinking, licentiousness, gambling, and smoking.

xin 心 Heart: One of the Three Realms and at the same time one of the Four Great Realms, in which context it is also known as the Realm of Emotional Suffering.

xin 信 Integrity: One of the Five Virtues, associated with Earth and the Spleen.

xinshi 信實 Integrity and Trust: The manifestation of Virtue associated with Earth and the Spleen.

xing 性 Inner Nature: One of the Three Realms. This is further subdivided into the Heavenly Nature *tianxing*, Habitual Nature *xixing*, and Inherited Nature *bingxing*.

yi 意 Intention: One of the Four Great Realms, also known as the Realm of Consciousness or the Paradise Level.

yi 義 Righteousness: One of the Five Virtues, associated with Metal and the Lung.

yinming 陰命 Yin Destiny: One of the three types of Destiny, associated with the Body and manifesting in the Inherited Nature (*bingxing*).

yinguo 因果 Cause and Effect: A technical term from Buddhism that explains the Karmic relationship between actions and their results, whether playing out within a single lifetime or passed on from previous ones.

yuan 怨 Blame: One of the Five Poisons, associated with Earth and the Spleen.

zhi 志 Commitment: One of the Four Great Realms, also known as the Realm of Enlightenment or the Buddha Level.

zhi 智 Wisdom: One of the Five Virtues, associated with Water and the Kidney.

zhong 忠 Loyalty: One of the key Confucian virtues.

zhuyi 主意 Firmness of Purpose: The manifestation of Virtue associated with Wood and the Liver.

zuishen 罪身 Body of Transgressions: One of the three aspects of the Body.

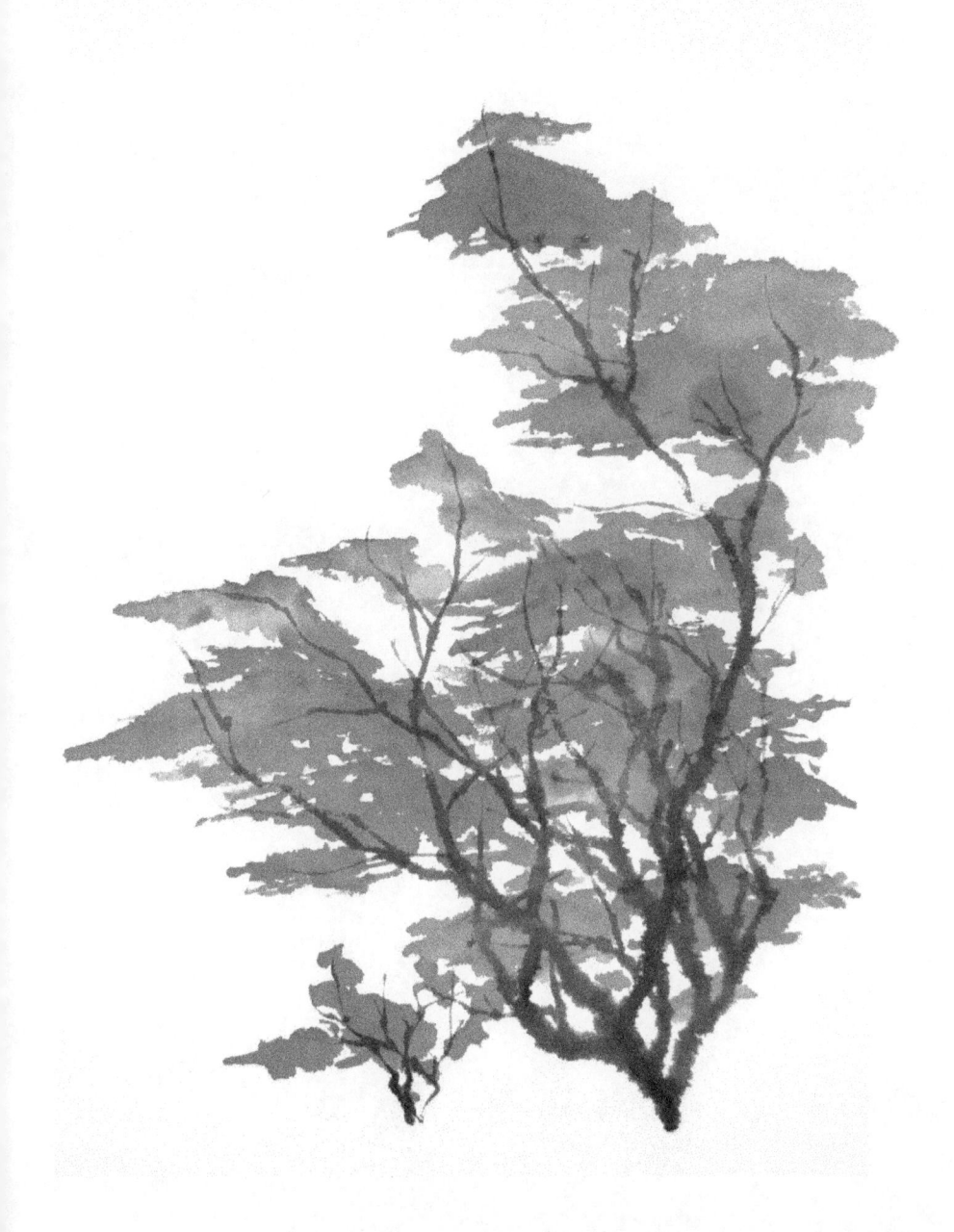

CPSIA information can be obtained
at www.ICGtesting.com
Printed in the USA
BVHW030829050719
552240BV00042B/259/P